Other Books By Tom Bisio

A Tooth From The Tiger's Mouth: *How to Treat Your Injuries with Powerful Healing Secrets of the Ancient Chinese Warriors*

Strategy and Change: *An Examination of Military Strategy, The I Ching and Ba Gua Zhang*

The Essentials of Ba Gua Zhang
By Gao Ji Wu and Tom Bisio

The Attacking Hands of Ba Gua Zhang
By Gao Ji Wu with Tom Bisio

Zheng Gu Tui Na: *A Chinese Medical Massage Textbook*
By Tom Bisio and Frank Butler

Nei Gong: The Authentic Classic. *A Translation of the Nei Gong Zhen Chuan* Translated by Tom Bisio, Huang Guo-Qi and Joshua Paynter

Ba Gua Circle Walking Nei Gong:
The Meridian Opening Palms of Ba Gua Zhang

by Tom Bisio

Outskirts Press, Inc.
Denver, Colorado

The opinions expressed in this manuscript are solely the opinions of the author and do not represent the opinions or thoughts of the publisher. The author has represented and warranted full ownership and/or legal right to publish all the materials in this book.

Ba Gua Circle Walking Nei Gong:
The Meridian Opening Palms of Ba Gua Zhang
All Rights Reserved.
Copyright © 2012
by Tom Bisio V1.0

This book may not be reproduced, transmitted, or stored in whole or in part by any means, including graphic, electronic, or mechanical without the express written consent of the publisher except in the case of brief quotations embodied in critical articles and reviews.

Outskirts Press, Inc.
http://www.outskirtspress.com

ISBN: 978-1-4327-9689-1

Outskirts Press and the "OP" logo are trademarks belonging to Outskirts Press, Inc.

PRINTED IN THE UNITED STATES OF AMERICA

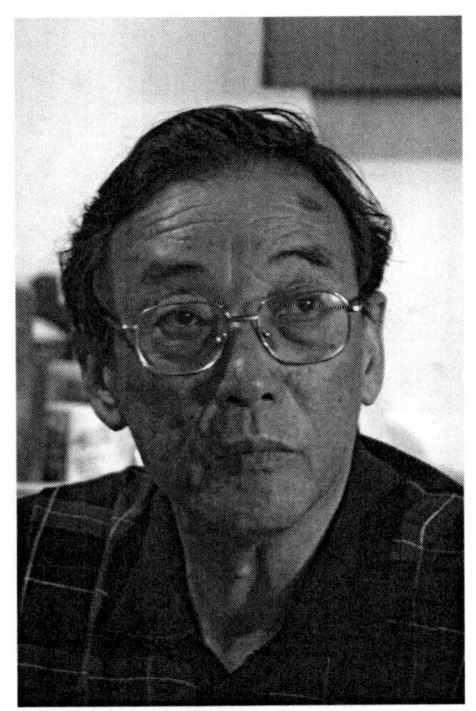

赵大元
Zhao Da Yuan

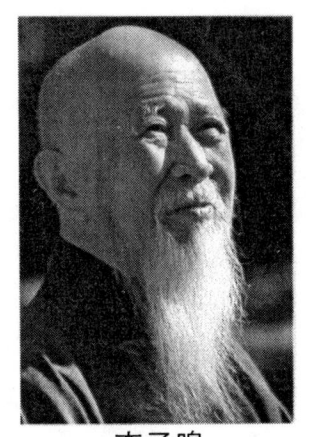

李子鳴
Li Zi Ming

This book is dedicated to Zhao Da Yuan and his teacher Li Zi Ming for their efforts and dedication in preserving and passing on the art of Ba Gua Zhang

My deep appreciation and thanks to Zhang Hua Sen, Wang Shi Tong and Gao Ji Wu for their patient teaching and open sharing of their knowledge of Ba Gua and Circle Walking Nei Gong.

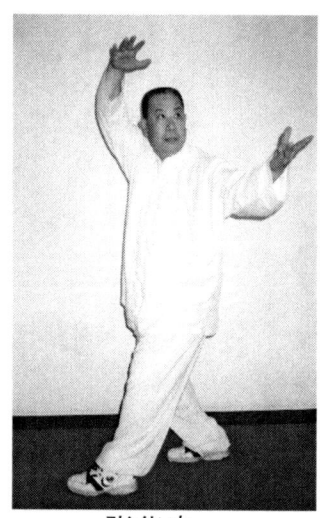

张华森
Zhang Hua Sen

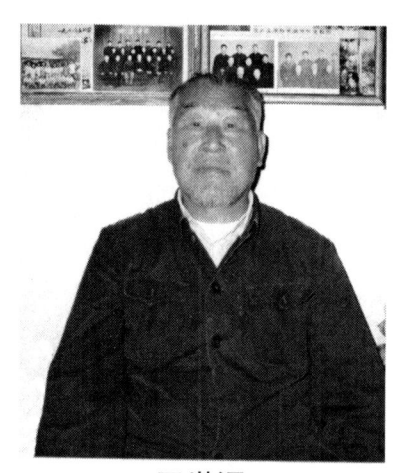

王世通
Wang Shi Tong

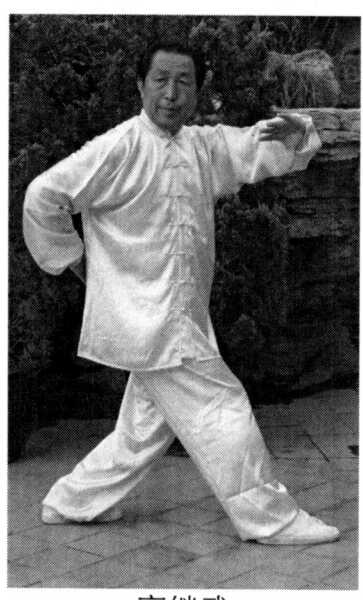

高继武
Gao Ji Wu

Acknowledgements

Endless thanks to my wife Valerie Ghent for her amazing photos of Gao Ji Wu and her ongoing collaboration on books, photos, videos and articles without which so many projects relating to Ba Gua Zhang simply would not happen. Some of the photos for the book were taken by Valerie and she did the final proofreading. Thank you Valerie for always being there to listen to my ideas and supporting me in these kinds of projects

Without Huang Guo Qi, my good friend of many years, so much of my understanding of the Chinese martial arts would not even be possible. Thank you Huang for all your work, help and friendship.

My thanks to Finbar McGrath for taking some of the photos from which drawings were rendered and for the thankless job of proofreading. Finbar and I also engaged in animated discussions about meridians and Nei Gong and these conversations also helped to shape the book.

My thanks to Zhao Da Yuan for sharing his knowledge with me.

My gratitude to Vince Black for setting my feet on the path.

This publication contains the ideas and opinions of the author. It is intended to provide helpful and informative material on the subjects addressed in the publication. It is sold with the understanding that the author and publisher are not engaged in rendering, or recommending medical, health or any other kind of personal professional services in the book. The reader should consult his or her medical, health or other competent professional before adopting any suggestions in the book or drawing inferences from it.

The author and publisher disclaim specifically disclaim all responsibility for any liability, loss, or risk, personal or otherwise, which in incurred as a consequence, directly or indirectly, of the use and application of the contents of this book.

Contents

Preface	1
How To Use This Book	3
Resources	6

Chapter 1
The Perfect Exercise: Ba Gua Circle Walking Nei Gong — 7

The Origin of Ba Gua Zhang	7
Walking as Exercise	8
Qi Gong and Nei Gong Benefit of Internal Exercise	9
Meditation	11
Breathing	12
Circle Walking Nei Gong	13

Chapter 2
Internal Exercise and Internal Martial Arts — 17

Nei Jia	17
Triads	17
Internal and External Martial Arts	18
Internal and External Exercise	19
The Six Harmonies	20
The Concept of Qi	23
The Purpose of Internal Martial Arts	25
Fundamental Forces: Water and Fire	26
The Nei Gong Triad	28
Opening the Meridians	31

Chapter 3
Jing Luo: The Meridian System — 33

Meridians	33
Acu-points	35
The Meridian System	36
Yin and Yang Channels	38
The Channels and Collaterals	39
The Meridians and the Fascia	41

Chapter 4
Ding Shi Ba Gua Nei Gong: Basic Alignments and Body Patterns — 45

Ding Shi and Circle Walking	45
The Downward Sinking Palm	48
Downward Sinking Palm: Stationary Practice	48

Linear Mud Stepping: The Slow Walk	49
General Body Alignments in Walking the Circle	56

Chapter 5
Walking The Circle — 63
Kou Bu and Bai Bu: Hooking and Swinging Steps	63
Walking the Circle in the Downward Sinking Palm Pattern	66

Chapter 6
The Eight Palms of Ding Shi — 73
Kidney Breathing	73
The Magpie Bridges	75
The Lao Gong Point	75
Changing Direction on the Circle: An Alternative Method	76
The Eight Ding Shi Palms	77
Downward Sinking Palm	78
Heaven Upholding Palm	81
Moon Embracing Palm	85
Ball Rolling Palm	88
Spear Upholding Palm	91
Heaven Pointing Ground Drawing Palm	93
Yin Yang Fish Palm	96
Millstone Pushing Palm	99
Peach Offering Palm	102

Chapter 7
The Six Yin and Yang Axes — 105
The Six Axes: Twelve Primary Channels	105
The Three Movements: Open, Close and Pivot	109
Taiyang	112
Shaoyang	114
Yangming	116
Taiyin	118
Shaoyin	120
Jueyin	122
Interaction of the Six Axes	124
Five Phases and Six Axes	125
The First Energetic Unit: Taiyin & Yangming	127
The Second First Energetic Unit: Shaoyin & Taiyang	129
The Third Energetic Unit: Jueyin & Shaoyang	131

The Eight Trigrams and the Five Elements   133

Chapter 8
The Eight Extraordinary Channels   135

    The Eight Extraordinary Channels   135
    General Functions of The Eight Extraordinary Vessels   136
    Nei Gong and The Extraordinary Vessels   137
    The Micro-Cosmic Orbit and The Extraordinary Vessels   140
    One Qi and One Breath   142
    Du Mai (Governing Vessel)   144
    Ren Mai (Conception Vessel)   148
    Chong Mai (Thrusting Vessel)   150
    Dai Mai (Belt Vessel)   154
    Yang Qiao Mai and Yin Qiao Mai (Heel Vessels)   157
    Yin Wei Mai and Yang Wei Mai (Linking Vessels)   163
    The Eight Psychic Channels   170

Chapter 9
The Eight Ding Shi Palms: Opening the Meridians   175

    The Eight Ding Shi Palms and the Meridians   175
    Kan and Li: Water and Fire   177
    Using the Eight Ding Shi to Open and Stimulate the Jing Luo   179
    Body Unity   180
    Downward Sinking Palm   182
    Moon Embracing Palm   185
    Heaven Upholding Palm   188
    Ball Rolling Palm   190
    Spear Upholding Palm   192
    Heaven Pointing Ground Drawing Palm   195
    Yin Yang Fish Palm   198
    Millstone Pushing Palm   202
    Peach Offering Palm   207

Chapter 10
Constitution and Illness: Adjusting Your Practice   209

    Sample Prescriptions   210
    Signs and Symptoms of Channel Disharmonies   212
    Signs and Symptoms of the Six Yin Yang Axes   212
        Taiyang   212
        Shaoyang   213
        Yangming   214

Taiyin	215
Shaoyin	216
Jueyin	217
Signs and Symptoms of the Eight Extraordinary Channels	218
Du Mai	218
Ren Mai	219
Chong Mai	219
Dai Mai	220
Yang Wei Mai	221
Yin Wei Mai	221
Yang Qiao Mai	222
Yin Qiao Mai	222

Chapter 11
Advanced Walking Patterns — 223

Figure Eight Pattern	223
The Yin Yang Winding Step: Method #1	224
The Yin Yang Winding Step: Method #2	225
Nine Palace Circle Walking Pattern	228

Chapter 12
The Ba Gua Energy Accepting Palm — 233

The Healing Power of Plants and Trees	233
Properties of Trees	234
Properties of Flowers	235
The Ba Gua Energy Accepting Palm	235

Bibliography — 241

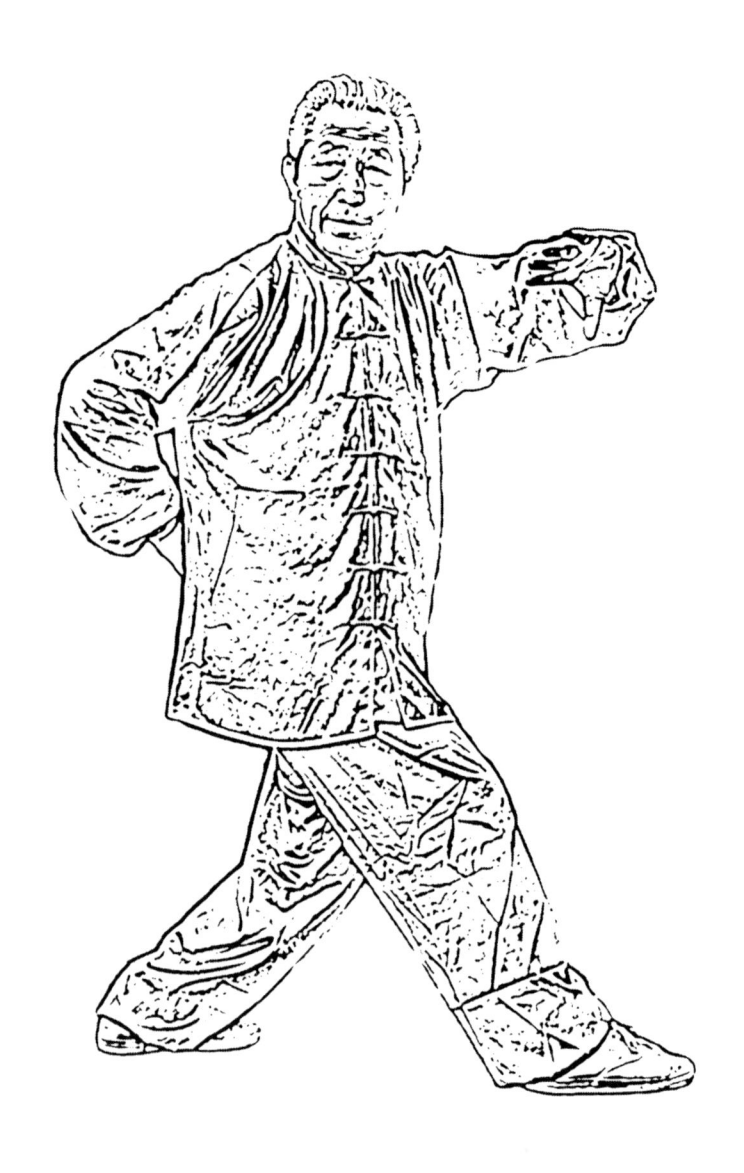

Yin Yang Fish Palm
Drawing from a photo of Gao Ji Wu taken by Valerie Ghent

Preface

In 2009 I met with Zhao Da Yuan, a well known Ba Gua master in Beijing. Zhao Da Yuan himself studied with Li Zi Ming one of the most famous masters in Beijing and a third generation exponent of Ba Gua. Zhao Da Yuan is well known for his ability to employ Ba Gua as a martial art and for his mastery of *qinna* (capture and seizing skills) which includes joint locks, seizing tendons, and striking vital points. However, Zhao Da Yuan is also a strong proponent of Ba Gua Zhang as a method of health preservation and nourishing life (*yang sheng*). During our meeting, Zhao explained to me that the Ba Gua training method of circular walking while holding specific postures (*Ding Shi Ba Gua Zhang*) benefited the meridians and internal organs in very specific ways. Each posture stimulates a different meridian or group of meridians. Therefore the practice of *Ding Shi* has profound effects on the body's organs and energy systems. Moreover, Zhao made it clear that understanding the specifics of the circle walking practice in relationship to the meridians allows one to adjust the practice of *Ding Shi* to specific individuals and their unique constitutional requirements. Zhao himself teaches students to alter their practice according to both general constitutional factors as well as specific health issues that may be occurring in the moment.

As our 2009 meeting was brief, Zhao Da Yuan did not have time to explain to me the details of the how the *Ding Shi* postures relate to the meridians. In May, 2011, I returned to Beijing and visited with Zhao again. This time I was able to receive from him the full explanation of the *Ding Shi* and their physical and energetic relationship to the meridians and organs of the body. Zhao is a clear and precise teacher. His remarks were punctuated by demonstrations and many examples to clarify important points. We also examined his hand-written notes from Li Zi Ming's personal instruction on *Ding Shi Ba Gua Zhang* in the early 1980's. This discussion and Li Zi Ming's notes form the basis of this book.

As a practitioner of traditional Chinese medicine and Nei Gong I found Zhao's discussion fascinating, especially as it confirmed many of the sensations I had felt while practicing Ba Gua. His transmission of this information reinforced to me the profound insights into health, the human body, and life that can be gleaned through the study Chinese medicine and the internal arts. I cannot emphasize enough the importance of "feeling" the meridians and their interconnections rather than understanding them only through books. It is my personal opinion that the meridians in general, and in particular the Eight Extraordinary Vessels, were originally understood through internal practices. Later these discoveries were written down and fixed to the very discrete pathways that appear in modern books. This also helps to explain the discrepancies between the channel pathways as they appear in Chinese medical texts and as they are described in Meditation and Nei Gong practices.

For those readers who are Ba Gua practitioners, I hope this book will enhance your understanding of the art of Ba Gua Zhang and its ability to promote health and vitality. Every senior master of Ba Gua Zhang that I have met emphasized to me the importance of the life nourishing, health promoting aspects of the art and felt that these facets of the art were of equal or even greater importance than the self-defense aspects.

Tom Bisio
New York City 2012

How to Use This Book

If you already practice Ba Gua circle walking you can simply incorporate the information contained in this book into your practice. If you have never practiced Ba Gua before and wish to use this book as a guide to learning and practicing Ba Gua Circle Walking Nei Gong, I suggest the following step-by-step approach.

Weeks 1 and 2

Start by accustoming yourself to the body alignments by holding the Downward Sinking Palm Posture for a minute or two on each side as though you are in the middle of a step. Then practice The Slow Walk exercise. Perform 10 steps - five steps on each side - taking a full minute or more to complete each individual step. Both the body alignments for Circle walking Nei Gong and the slow walking exercise are described in Chapter 4. Specific alignments for the Downward Sinking Palm are reiterated in Chapter 6.

Weeks 3 and 4

Continue to practice the slow walk for 10 minutes, but now add the basic circle walking described in Chapter 5 – still using the Downward Sinking Palm body pattern. The walking speed will be smoother and quicker than in The Slow Walk exercise, perhaps taking 30 seconds to walk 8 steps. Start with a circle that takes 8-12 steps to complete and walk. In the beginning it can be useful to count either the steps or the circle:

1. Walk 64 steps in one direction (8 circles) – about two to three minutes.
2. Change direction using the 4 step turn (Chapter 5).
3. Walk 64 steps in the other direction (8 circles).
4. Repeat this 3-4 times.

Weeks 5 and 6

You can continue to practice the slow walk or transition to just walking the circle. Often it is useful to split the training by practicing the slow walk in one training session and later in the day practicing circle walking. Now add the Heaven Uplifting palm to your practice.

1. Walk 64 steps in one direction holding the Downward Sinking Palm Posture (8 circles or 2-3 minutes).
2. Change direction using the 4 step turn (chapter 5).
3. Walk 64 steps in the other direction holding the Downward Sinking Palm Posture (8 circles).
4. Repeat this 3-4 times.
5. Repeat steps 1-4 holding the Heaven Uplifting Palm.

Beyond 6 Weeks

From this point on you can slowly add the other postures, at first practicing them in the order presented. However, the Fruit Offering Palm is often practiced as the second posture – it serves as a transition between the Downward Sinking Palm and the Heaven Uplifting Palm.

A 36-minute training session would consist of performing each of the nine postures for 2 minutes in each direction. Of course one can walk longer in each posture if time permits.

Important: Circle walking Nei Gong can be difficult and uncomfortable in the beginning as it realigns the knees, ankles and hips so that they move correctly with spiraling forces. Start slowly and don't push the body too hard in the beginning. Listen to your body and if there is pain, reassess the body alignments – often there is a small error in the stepping.

Later the advanced walking patterns can be added and one can practice flowing freely between the different postures.

Tips for Practice
- Keep the body loose and relaxed when walking the circle. Slowly build up the length of the training time or the number of circles you walk so that you can walk comfortably without straining the body.
- The intention and posture guide the breath and the qi to the meridians, organs and tissues, but the intention should be applied gently and naturally so that nothing is forced. If the mind and intention are forced, the qi can block and the meridians will not open and flow freely.
- The basic practice method (walking the circle holding all nine postures in a single session) naturally balances, strengthens and regulates the body.
- If you are not familiar with diagnosis in traditional Chinese medicine you should consult with a qualified practitioner of Chinese medicine before modifying the basic practice method to address medical or health issues.
- When modifying your practice to adjust for illness or imbalance, it is important to keep in mind that the goal is to return to the normal, balanced practice method once the body has returned to a state of balance.

Resources:

The resources below can provide you with more information on Ba Gua, Ba Gua Circle Walking Nei Gong, Internal Exercise, and traditional Chinese medicine.

Video footage of the Ba Gua Circle Walking Nei Gong is available on the Internal Arts International (IAI) and New York Internal Arts (NYIA) websites and in the Ba Gua Concepts, Vol. 1 Video.

Websites:

Internal Arts International (www.internalartsinternational.com)

New York Internal Arts (internalartsinternational.com)

Articles, books, videos and downloadable information on Chinese Internal Arts, traditional Chinese medicine, Nei Gong and Life Nourishing (*Yang Shen*) practices

- Seminars, classes on Ba Gua Zhang, Xing Yi Quan and Nei Gong
- Online Ba Gua lessons from masters in China
- Online Academy for Ba Gua Zhang

DVDs:

Single Step Productions Ba Gua Concepts Series

Ba Gua Concepts Vol. 1: Ding Shi

Ba Gua Concepts Vol. 2: Lao Ba Zhang & Linear Applications

Ba Gua Concepts Vol. 3: Swimming Body Ba Gua Chain Linking Form

Available at: http://www.singlestepproductions.com/

Books:

Essential Anatomy for Healing and Martial Arts by Marc Tedeschi (Weatherhill inc., 2000) features detailed drawings and photographs of the meridians and acu-points. It is very useful adjunct to understanding the concepts presented in this book.

Chapter 1
The Perfect Exercise: Ba Gua Circle Walking Nei Gong

The Origin of Ba Gua Nei Gong

The primary internal exercise in Ba Gua Zhang (Eight Diagram Palm) is to walk in a circle holding fixed postures. This practice is known as *Ding Shi Ba Gua Zhang*. It is believed that Dong Hai Chuan, the founder of Ba Gua Zhang, synthesized the best of various martial styles in order to create Ba Gua. However the key element of this new style was the practice of walking in a circle while holding various postures that energize and strengthen the body while calming the mind and refining and purifying the spirit. It is believed that Dong studied with the Dragon Gate school of Daoism which practiced a form of Daoist circle walking meditation whose purpose was to open and harmonize the meridians of the body in order to promote health and focus and quiet the mind. Daoist practitioners used this practice, called "Rotating in the Worship of Heaven," not for martial purposes, but to refine qi and spirit through external movement in order to realize internal stillness or emptiness (ie: the Dao). Purportedly Dong saw that this circle walking had value, not only as a meditation and health exercise, but also as the foundation of an effective method of martial arts.[1] As a result the following statement is attributed to Dong Hai Chuan:

Training in martial arts ceaselessly is inferior to walking the circle;
In Ba Gua Zhang circle walking practice is the font of all training.

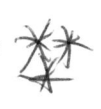

---

[1] *The Origins of Pa Kua Chang - Part 3,* by Dan Miller. Pa Kua Chang Journal Vol. 3, No. 4 May/June 1993. Pacific Grove, CA: High View Publications, p. 27

Walking as Exercise

Modern research has only recently confirmed something that the Chinese clearly knew over a thousand years ago – that regular, moderate exercise enhances resistance to disease, improves emotional well-being and reduces the incidence and risk of high blood pressure, stroke and diseases like diabetes. Studies have shown that a moderate exercise like walking may actually produce greater results than more intensive cardio-vascular exercise. As proof, some doctors point to the work of Hiroshi Nose:

> *Hiroshi Nose, M.D., Ph.D., a professor of sports medical sciences at Shinshu University Graduate School of Medicine in Japan, who has enrolled thousands of older Japanese citizens in an innovative, five-month-long program of brisk, interval-style walking (three minutes of fast walking, followed by three minutes of slower walking, repeated 10 times). The results have been striking. "Physical fitness — maximal aerobic power and thigh muscle strength — increased by about 20 percent," [Dr. Nose wrote in an e-mail], "which is sure to make you feel about 10 years younger than before training." The walkers' "symptoms of lifestyle-related diseases (hypertension, hyperglycemia and obesity) decreased by about 20 percent," he added, while their depression scores dropped by half.*[2]

Other researchers have shown that walking aids in controlling weight. A 15-year study found that middle-aged women who walked for at least an hour a day were able to maintain their weight. Those who did not walk gained weight. *In addition, a recent seminal study found that when older people started a regular program of brisk walking, the volume of their*

---

[2] *What's the Single Best Exercise?* by Gretchen Reynolds Published: April 15, 2011
New York Times Magazine ttp://www.nytimes.com/2011/04/17/magazine/mag-17exercise-t.html

hippocampus, a portion of the brain involved in memory, increased significantly.[3]

Walking is also superior to many other forms of exercise, as it balances the musculature of the legs and utilizes the entire body through the natural oppositional movements of the arms and legs and their concomitant production of spiral movements through the torso, which in turn relaxes the diaphragm and engages the inter-costal and stomach muscles. This in turn stimulates the organs of digestion and improves circulation throughout the entire body.

Qi Gong and Nei Gong: The Benefit of Internal Exercise

Internal Exercises like Qi Gong and Nei Gong, and martial arts like Tai Ji Quan, which feature slow deliberate movements performed in conjunction with deep breathing and focused mind-intention, have been shown to produce a multitude of improvements in physiological functioning and resistance to disease:

- One study showed that Qi Gong exercise increased blood flow to the brain, creating improvements in symptoms such as memory, dizziness, and insomnia.[4]
- A study of people with high blood pressure showed that after 12 weeks of Qi Gong, blood pressure and cholesterol levels were lower.
- A study in Korea indicated that regular practice of Qi Gong reduced blood pressure, as well as reduced cortisol levels. Cortisol is

---

[3] Ibid.
[4] *Anti-Aging Benefits of Qigong,* by Kenneth Sancier Ph. D., http://www.qigonginstitute.org/html/papers/Anti-Aging_Benefits_of_Qigong.html

produced by the adrenal gland and is often referred to as the "stress hormone" as it is involved in response to stress.[5]

- In the treatment of asthma, self-applied Qi Gong led to significant cost decreases such as reduction in sick days, hospitalization days, emergency consultations, respiratory tract infections and the number of drugs and drug costs.[6]

- Unfavorable changes of sex hormone levels due to aging were retarded by regular practice of Qi Gong exercises.

- Superoxide dismutase (SOD), an anti-aging enzyme that is produced naturally by the body, declines with age. SOD is believed to destroy free radicals that may cause aging. In one study the SOD levels of retired workers who did Qi Gong exercises showed that the mean level of SOD was increased by Qi Gong exercise.[7]

- A study sponsored by the National Institute on Aging and National Center for Complementary and Alternative Medicine compared the effects of Qi Gong and Tai Chi on adults 60 and older, measuring their immunity to the Varicella Zoster Virus that causes shingles. After 12 weeks, the participants had raised their immunity to the virus.

- Regular practice of Qi Gong can improve sleep and reduce daytime fatigue and drowsiness.

- Qi Gong and Tai Chi have been shown to reduce stress and psychological distress.

---

[5] *Qigong Reduced Blood Pressure and Catecholamine Levels of Patients with Essential Hypertension,* by Myung-Suk Lee, Myeong Soo Lee et als 2003, Vol. 113, No. 12, Pages 1691-1701. http://informahealthcare.com/doi/abs/10.1080/00207450390245306
[6] *Multifaceted Health Benefits of Medical Qigong,* by Kenneth M. Sancier, Ph.D. and Devatara Holman MS, MA, Lac J. Alt Compl Med. 2004; 10(1):163-166.
[7] *Anti-Aging Benefits of Qigong,* by Kenneth Sancier Ph.D., http://www.qigonginstitute.org/html/papers/Anti-Aging_Benefits_of_Qigong.html

- The practice of Qi Gong has been shown to reduce arthritis pain and stiffness in the joints. Regular practice of Qi Gong helped patients reduce their pain medication.[8]
- A clinical trial at Tufts Medical Center found that after 12 weeks of Tai Ji Quan, patients with Fibromyalgia, did significantly better in measurements of pain, fatigue, physical functioning, sleeplessness and depression than a comparable group given stretching exercises and wellness education. Patients who practiced Tai Ji Quan were also more likely to sustain improvement three months later.[9]

Meditation

The practice of Qi Gong and Nei Gong also involve control of the breath and the cultivation of a calm, relaxed mind that puts aside distracting thoughts for the duration of the practice session. This has been labeled "the relaxation response" by researchers like Herbert Benson. Benson found that this mind-body state, common to various methods of meditation and exercises like Qi Gong and Nei Gong, could counteract the harmful effects of stress and the "flight or fight" response. Many of the following conditions can be significantly improved or cured when people regularly engage in a practice that produces the "relaxation response":[10]

- Constipation
- Cardiac Arrhythmia
- Herpes Simplex

---

[8] *Effects of Qigong Therapy on Arthritis*: A Review and Report of a Pilot Trial by Kevin W Chen and Tianjun Liu. Medical Paradigm: June 2004 - Volume 1, Number 1.; www.wishus.org/researchpapers/Arthritis.pdf

[9] *Tai Chi Reported to Ease Fibromyalgia,* by Pam Belluck. The New York Times, August 18, 2010. http://www.nytimes.com/2010/08/19/health/19taichi.html

[10] *The Relaxation Response,* By Herbert Benson MD, New York: HarperCollins, 2000. First Published in 1975 by William Morrow and Co. Inc. pp. xli-xlii.

- Bronchial Asthma
- Diabetes
- Duodenal Ulcers
- Hypertension
- Insomnia
- Pain

More recently researchers reported that those who meditated for about 30 minutes a day for eight weeks had measurable changes in gray-matter density in parts of the brain associated with memory, sense of self, empathy and stress. M.R.I. brain scans taken before and after the participants' meditation regimen found increased gray matter in the hippocampus, an area important for learning and memory. The images also showed a reduction of gray matter in the amygdala, a region connected to anxiety and stress.[11]

Breathing

The slow rhythmic deep abdominal breathing common to Qi Gong and Nei Gong exercises is also an important element in their efficacy in promoting health and resistance to disease. Breathing "is" life. While we can go without food and water for days, we cannot go without breathing for even a few minutes. This most basic life rhythm has profound effects on the whole human organism. The movements of the diaphragm and ribs in inhalation and exhalation help the vena cava to return blood to the heart. Additionally, the organs of digestion have direct and indirect attachments to the diaphragm, whose piston-like action in breathing aids digestion and

---

[11] *How Meditation May Change the Brain*, by Sindya N. Bhanoo January 28, 2011, New York Times http://well.blogs.nytimes.com/2011/01/28/how-meditation-may-change-the-brain/

peristalsis. Even the kidneys move slightly with every breath. It is no surprise that impaired breathing can have profound affects on the functioning of the internal organs. It has been clinically shown that slow, even breathing at a rate of less than ten breaths per minute can modulate blood pressure. Regular practice of slowed breathing actually produced a drop in blood pressure of 20-30 points. The FDA has approved biofeedback-like devices that aid patients in slowing their breathing in order to treat hypertension. Other benefits of slow, relaxed, deep breathing include reduced incidence of asthma and bronchitis as well as increased lung capacity and stamina.

Circle Walking Nei Gong

Ding Shi Ba Gua Zhang (the Nei Gong practice associated with the martial art Ba Gua Zhang) is unique as it combines the benefits of walking with the internal movements and deep abdominal breathing of Nei Gong and Qi Gong practices, as well as the relaxed and calm mind-intention associated with meditation and the relaxation response. Zhao Da Yuan feels that the element that makes circle walking "internal" is the link between mind and body that is forged during the circle walk practice. Zhao and other Ba Gua practitioners believe that engaging the mind-intention with the body movements neuro-muscularly reprograms the body to work more efficiently by firing the right muscles at the right moment. This not only reduces inefficiency, but also optimizes the strength fluidity of the body.

Zhao explains that when the average person contracts a muscle, 45 to 50 percent of the muscle fibers in that muscle "fire." A trained athlete, or a person who repetitively works a set of muscles performing a certain task, may contract about 70 percent of the muscle fiber in a given muscle for a given purpose. His theory is that if the practitioner holds a static upper body posture with focused concentration for an extended period of time, as in the circle walk practice, he or she will be able to develop the ability to get more muscle fibers to contract at the same time for the same purpose. Holding a static posture for an extended period of time, or moving very slowly as in Tai Ji Quan, a more complete physical development occurs than in exercises where the body moves rapidly. Secondary muscles are conditioned and the body learns to act in an integrated and unified fashion.[12]

Practitioners like Zhao Da Yuan and his teacher Li Zi Ming feel that Ba Gua is the ultimate Nei Gong exercise because it is the culmination of a tradition of Dao Yin (guiding, pulling and leading qi exercises), Tu Na (breathing exercises), Nei Gong (internal exercises), martial arts, Daoist meditation, Daoist alchemical practices, and other *Yang Sheng* (Life Nourishing) practices that date back at least as far as the early Han dynasty. Because of the relatively late development of Ba Gua Zhang as a martial art (the founder, Dong Hai Chuan, lived from 1813 to 1882), Ba Gua draws on all of these traditions and, according to some experts, incorporated the best methods from these various traditions into its techniques and training methods.

Both Zhao Da Yuan and Li Zi Ming feel that the circle walking practice of Ding Shi Ba Gua Zhang conforms more completely with the intrinsic movement of the universe and the natural world than other forms of exercise. By moving constantly and changing postures and directions, one is more in harmony with nature which is itself always changing and moving. Zhao Da Yuan feels that this makes it easier for the mind to achieve the

---

[12] http://pakuachangjournal.com/circleWalk.php?page=6

empty mind that is characteristic of the meditative state. To paraphrase Li Zi Ming:

> *The movements of the celestial bodies in the universe contain both rotation and circulation. The human body is microcosm of the universe – a small heavenly circle. The theory of Ba Gua draws upon this observation of the heavenly bodies by using rotation and circulation through its walking and turning practice. This practice harmonizes the practitioner with the natural movement of qi of the universe. Ba Gua's practice of walking and rotating therefore conforms to the natural principle of the world around us. By walking the circle and rotating the body, qi is aroused and circulates inside the body. This in turn strengthens the body, improves circulation and resistance to disease, and improves the functioning of the respiratory and digestive systems. Additionally it produces a unified strength that stems from the arousal of the qi. This strength can then be employed in the martial arts.*[13]

Walking the circle as a Ba Gua Nei Gong practice is not simply walking. It combines the benefits of walking with Qi Gong and meditation. It also develops a refined strength that can be employed in martial arts and other physical activities. As the body turns, and rotates, the muscles, fascia and energy pathways of the body (the meridians) are stimulated by spiraling actions that engage the whole body. The deep abdominal breathing combines with the body alignments to connect the lower body to the waist and upper limbs so that the whole body can be sensed. Inside, the mind is quiet and observant, while outside there is movement and rotation. This

---

[13] *A Brief Introduction to the Body Strengthening Function of the Eight Diagram Palm Qi Gong* by Li Zi Ming, Translated by Huang Guo Qi, Pa Kua Chang Journal Vol. 5 No. 1 Nov./Dec. 1994, Pacific Grove CA: High View Publications pp. 17-19.

creates a refined strength that is combined with internal relaxation, akin to the natural and relaxed strength of a cat. Perhaps this is why Ba Gua practitioners place such a premium on walking. Li Zi Ming summarized the importance of walking, and in particular, Ba Gua Circle Walking Nei Gong by simply saying:

> **Hundreds of exercises are not as good as simply walking;**
> **Walking is the master of hundreds of exercises.**[14]

---

[14] *Liang Zhen Pu Eight Diagram Palm* by Li Zi Ming; translated by Huang Guo Qi and compiled and edited by Vince Black. Pacific Grove, CA: High View Publications, 1993, p. 21.

Chapter 2
Internal Exercise and Internal Martial Arts

Nei Jia

Nei Jia 內家 literally means "inner family or inner school." When the character for "fist" is added - resulting in 內家拳 *Nei Jia Quan* – then the term refers specifically to styles of martial arts that in English we call "internal." Today these styles are considered to include Tai Ji Quan, Xing Yi Quan, Ba Gua Zhang, Tong Bei Quan, Yi Quan (Da Cheng Quan) and Liu Ho Ba Fa. Other styles are sometimes called "internal," including the Japanese art of Aikido. However, as the term *Nei Jia* is a Chinese concept, we must examine define and examine the *Nei Jia* in the context of Chinese martial arts. In fact, many teachers of internal martial arts never really say what an internal art is. This is because the nature of something internal is that it is sensed and experienced internally rather than perceived externally. Hence words are poor conveyers of what the concept "internal" actually means.

Triads

In this discussion, the idea of triads – groups of three – will be used to help understand the concept of internal. Triads are an important concept in Chinese thought. The most basic triad in Chinese philosophy is that of Heaven, Earth and Human Beings. This is most often depicted with Heaven above, Earth below and Human Beings in the center. This triad is the basis of *San Ti Shi* the "Trinity" posture, or Three Body Pattern in Xing Yi Quan (Form-Intention or Form-Image Boxing). From this triad, many other triads have been developed to explain internal arts and internal training. Heaven's energy (yang qi) flows downward and is received by Earth. Earth's energy (yin qi) flows upward. The two interact and co-mingle in living things. Earth manifests and upholds physical forms in response to Heaven's images. There is an interaction of form and intention, images and manifestations, qi and substance.

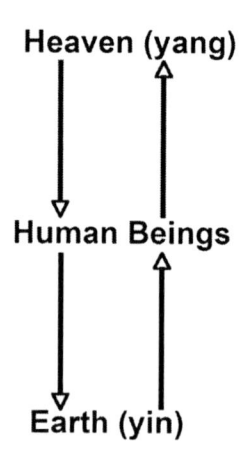

Heaven (yang)

↕

Human Beings

↕

Earth (yin)

Internal and External Martial Arts

At first glance, the primary difference between internal and external martial arts seems to be one of method. Speaking generally, the focus of internal arts is on principles rather than specific techniques. Internal arts have techniques, but from the very beginning it is understood that techniques are merely expressions of the principles and the ultimate goal is to create them in the moment out of the interaction of one's energy and intention with the opponent's energy and intention. Secondly, while generally speaking the external arts focus their training methods on developing muscular strength, speed and athletic prowess, internal arts stress relaxation, mind-intention, stillness and natural movement. Lastly, the internal arts use alignment, breath and structural dynamics to actualize the movement of the vital force through the channels and collaterals (*Jing Luo*) or meridians. This is said to cultivate "whole body power" which does not rely on muscular strength, speed and athleticism. This idea has considerable overlap with the idea of body mechanics – i.e.: bio-mechanical principles of movement that increase efficiency. However, as we shall see, the two concepts are not identical.

Internal

Principles

Relaxation; Mind-Intention

Alignment; Breath; Structure; Qi

External

Techniques

Muscular Strength; Speed; Athleticism

Body Mechanics; Bio-Mechanics

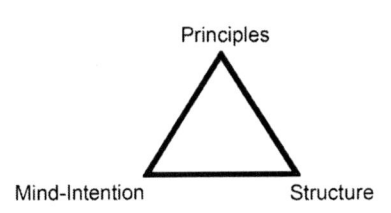

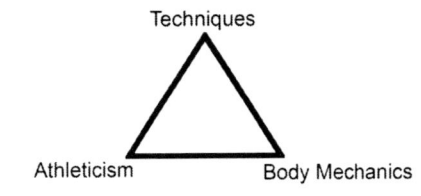

Internal
- Principles (top)
- Mind-Intention (bottom-left)
- Structure (bottom-right)

External
- Techniques (top)
- Athleticism (bottom-left)
- Body Mechanics (bottom-right)

Internal and External Exercise

One interesting way to look at these differentiations is by examining the concept of the "Three Harms" in the practice of Nei Gong. The three harms provide an excellent differentiation between "internal" exercise and "external" exercise. The three harms are:

1. Forced Breathing

   Forced Breathing can cause a stuffy, distended feeling in the chest and diaphragm. Forced breathing can also damage the lung qi. Breathing should be free, natural and unrestrained.

2. Labored Use of Strength

   Holding tension or power in a single part of the body in order to exert force. Not only does this break the feeling of connected, whole body movement, but it can lead to stagnation of qi and blood in local areas.

3. <u>Throwing Out the Chest & Sucking In the Abdomen</u>

This body alignment can lead to stasis of qi in the chest, so that the qi fails to descend to *Dantian*. The energy is blocked and cannot flow through the whole body. The qi floats upward so that the balance of the body is thrown off.

It is easy to see that the forced breath, panting and chest breathing that is a result of forcing the heart to work harder, as in aerobics and calisthenics, is the opposite of the breathing in Nei Gong exercises, in which the breathing occurs deep in the diaphragm ("Kidney Breathing"), and is slow, soft, long and even. Weight exercises and calisthenics which isolate muscle groups so that they can be worked to the maximum, or even to "failure," involve the labored use of strength as opposed to the whole body connected movement favored in internal exercise. Lastly, the over-developed chest and shoulders and washboard flat stomach favored by athletes and proponents of external exercise, is the antithesis of the relaxed chest and shoulders and rounded belly that result from performing internal exercises.

The Six Harmonies

Another pair of triads that internal martial arts practitioners often use to differentiate internal from external are the Six Harmonies – three internal and three external. The six harmonies discuss principles that are fundamental to internal exercise and internal martial arts.

Three External Harmonies

Harmony between Shoulder and Hip

Harmony between Elbow and Knee

Harmony between Hand and Foot

Three Internal Harmonies

Harmony between Mind and Intention (*Yi*)

Harmony between Intention (*Yi*) and Qi

Harmony between Qi and Power/Force (*Jin/Fa Jin; Li/ Fa Li*)

The shoulder and hip move together and support each other, as do the elbow and knee, and hand and foot. This means that these joints are linked and line up for efficient structure and power delivery. The shoulder is also considered to be the "root" of the arm, the elbow is the middle and the hand is the "tip". Similarly, the hip is the root, the knee is the middle and the foot is the tip. Power and force come from the root and manifest in the tip. In substance this is the same – or should be - in both internal and external exercise and martial arts. To some degree this is just a question of correct body mechanics.

The Internal Harmonies are a different matter. They must link with the three external harmonies in a seamless way. The mind-intention (*Yi*) guides the qi, which in turn actualizes force and power, which are themselves an emanation of the mind and intention. This is not as simple as deciding to do something with force and then doing it. Zhan Zhuang or "stake standing" is a good example. Standing or holding fixed postures is one of the fundamental exercises in internal martial arts. In holding the embrace posture for example, the body relaxes, the joints are aligned (external harmonies), and with the intention one guides the qi to the tips of the body so that qi fills the entire body. At the same time, there are oppositional forces operating in every direction which are not a product of bone, muscle and sinew but of the intention: The head and upper back erect upward while the tail sinks down, producing oppositional forces that pull

21

the spine in opposite directions. The arms feel like they are supporting and embracing inward, while at the same time the arms are pulling apart. Simultaneously throughout the body there is twisting, spiraling, wrapping inward and outward, extending and stretching, retracting, embracing, pulling apart and pushing together. These forces are manifestations of yin and yang, positive and negative – they are oppositional but also complimentary. They are balanced which minimizes body tension. All of this is a product of internal intention and internal "movement" occurring without visible (external) muscle tension or movement.

Additionally in holding postures or body patterns, whether they are Zhan Zhuang, San Ti Shi (in Xing Yi) or Ding Shi (in Ba Gua Zhang), there is an internal sensing going on. The oppositional and yet complimentary forces, allow one to sense the stillness within movement and the movement within stillness. Two equal and opposing forces produce no visible movement - they allow one to sense stillness. Yet within this stillness the forces are still operating – there is movement inside. As the body relaxes into the postures, one feels comfortable, at ease; the muscles relax and the bones seem to support while the muscles slacken and let go. Within this relaxation, this slackening, there is still force and strength, the product of the oppositional forces. Within the strength there is relaxation and flexibility. The body is not committed in any one direction; it is moving in all directions at the same time. Even though the body may feel still and appears to be still, there is a faint stirring of movement that is constantly in the process of being actualized.

The Concept of Qi

Qi is a concept integral to the internal harmonies and to the oppositional forces discussed above. But what is qi? There is no single word in the English language that adequately expresses the concept of qi. It can be translated to mean a gas or a vapor, or understood as electromagnetic waves or fields of force. The famous Chinese scholar Joseph Needham felt that the term: "Matter-Energy" might most appropriately express the idea of qi.[15] For simplicity, qi is often erroneously usually referred to as "Energy" or "Vital-Energy" in medical discussions. Webster's Dictionary defines "Energy" as follows:

- Vitality or affective force
- The capacity of acting, operating or producing an effect
- Inherent power
- Vigorousness
- Activity and the product or effect of activity
- The capacity for doing work or the equivalent as in a coiled spring (potential energy) or a speeding train.
- Having existence independent of matter (as light or X-rays traversing a vacuum)[16]

Qi is at the same time all and none of these things. To understand the concept of qi more clearly, it is helpful to study the ideogram itself and to look at how the Chinese have conceptualized qi throughout the centuries. The Chinese character for Qi depicts vapors curling and rising from the

---

[15] *The Shorter Science & Civilization in China: Vol 1,* Joseph Needham, Cambridge University Press, 1978. p.239.
[16] *Webster's 3rd New International Dictionary,* Springfield, Mass.: G&C : Merriman Co., 1961, p.751.

ground to form clouds above. The ancient oracle bone, bronze or seal form of the character depicts this very clearly:

Qi 气

Later the ideogram was expressed showing vapors rising to form a layer of clouds. This is also part of the character for steam:

Qi 气

The modern form of the character adds grain by using the character *mi* (rice) which is depicted as: 米. This creates an image of steam or vapor rising from cooking rice.

气 + 米 = 氣 Qi

Various interpretations may be made. The ideogram for qi may depict the nurturing energies of rice reduced to their smallest component, a vapor, or, as Needham indicated, the changing states of energy and matter.

In early Chinese Texts, qi is used to refer to various phenomena:

- Air
- Mists and Fog
- Moving Clouds
- Aromas
- Vapors
- Smoke
- Breathing – Inhalation and Exhalation

In common usage, qi can refer to air, gases and vapors, smells, spirit, vigor, morale, attitude, the emotions (particularly anger), as well as tone, atmospheric changes, the weather, breath and respiration. In the body *qi* is often discerned by its actions, *the balanced and orderly vitalities, partly derived from the air we breathe, that cause physical changes and maintain life.*[17] In Chinese medicine, when we say that someone is healthy, it is because the functioning of the their body, the physical manifestations of the their qi, are orderly and without dysfunction. Every movement, every thought and emotion, our metabolism, every movement of life and consciousness, is in some measure a manifestation of qi. Benjamin Schwartz adds an important element to the definition of qi when he says:

> *It is also clear, however that* qi *comes to embrace properties which we would call psychic, emotional, spiritual, numinous and even "mystical." It is precisely at this point that Western definitions of "matter" and the physical which systemically exclude these properties from their definition do not at all correspond to* qi.[18]

To sum up, qi is something that can be felt, internally sensed and understood, but it cannot be seen, measured or quantified. We sense qi and we can observe its manifestations and effects, but we cannot easily define it, so words often confuse the issue, which is why many teachers in the internal arts do not say much about qi. However, one should keep in mind that this reluctance to talk about qi, rather than negating its importance, actually underscores it.

The Purpose of Internal Martial Arts

Teachers of internal martial arts repeatedly say that the internal arts are not just for fighting and that approaching these arts with only this

---

[17] *Traditional Medicine in Contemporary China: Science, Medicine and Technology in East Asia Vol. 2,* by Nathan Sivin. Ann Arbor: Center for Chinese Studies University of Michigan, 1987. pp. 46-7.
[18] *The World of Thought in Ancient China* by Benjamin I. Schwartz, Cambridge, Mass: The Belknap press of Harvard University Press, 1985. p.181.

purpose in mind will ultimately lead to disappointment. Internal martial arts have three purposes which are expressed in the following triad:

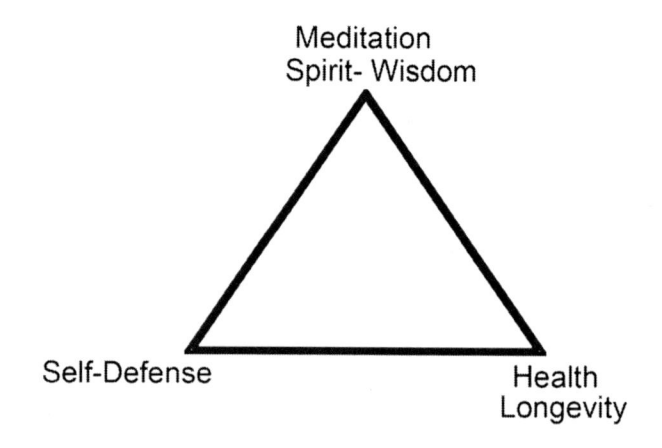

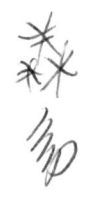

```
              Meditation
            Spirit- Wisdom
                 /\
                /  \
               /    \
              /      \
             /_____\
       Self-Defense    Health
                      Longevity
```

This requires a balanced approach to training:

- Breathing methods (*Tu Na*)
- Health exercises and Nei Gong
- Martial techniques
- Form and technique as an expression of principles
- Training in harmony with seasons
- Weapons as an extension of hand methods
- Training as meditation – stillness within movement and movement within stillness

Fundamental Forces: Water and Fire

On the most basic level, internal martial arts and internal exercises focus on engaging with the two fundamental forces in the body: water and fire, the archetypal expressions of yin and yang which move within human beings. These forces have a relationship with the kidneys (water) and the heart (fire). The *Yi Jing* trigrams, Water-Kan and Fire-Li are employed in martial arts, traditional medicine and in Daoist meditation as emblems or symbols of water and fire and the heart and kidneys.

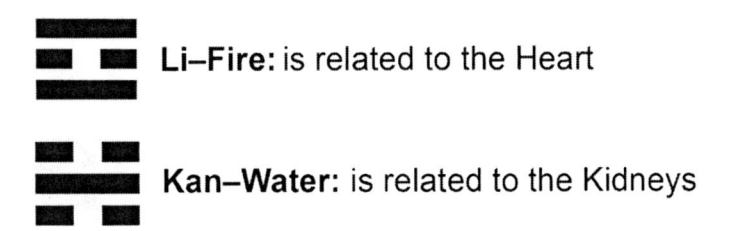

Li–Fire: is related to the Heart

Kan–Water: is related to the Kidneys

The fire of the heart communicates with the "moving qi between the kidneys," the *Mingmen* fire, the original fire that drives the human organism. The trigram Kan, which is associated with the water element in Chinese cosmology and the kidneys in Chinese medicine, is often used to represent the kidneys and *Mingmen*. Kan consists of two broken (yin) lines enclosing a single (yang) solid line. This yang line is Mingmen, the "moving qi" between the two kidneys, or the "hidden fire within water." Fire is balanced by water. Water has a tendency to sink downward and fire has a tendency to flare upward. In order for heart and kidneys to communicate, water and fire must commingle and inter-transform. This aids the interaction of *Jing* (essence) with the spirit of the heart, which manifests visibly in the light of consciousness that shines out of a person's eyes.

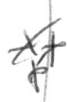

How does one aid the circulation and inter-transformation of Fire-Li and Water-Kan? In the internal arts, one of the functions of the Nei Gong postures and forms is to facilitate the interaction of Kan and Li. The trigrams are useful images in Nei Gong because they elucidate the relationship between the chest and the lower abdomen. Kan has a solid, yang line in the middle, so the lower abdomen (Dan Tian) is said to be "full" (of qi and breath) relative to the chest. Li has a broken line in the middle, so the chest is thought to be "empty" relative to the Dan Tian. These qualities attributed to Kan and Li are encapsulated in the following two statements which, when recited in Chinese, act as a kind of mnemonic:

1) Solid (substantial; full) abdomen, unimpeded chest. (*Shi Fu Chang Xiong*)

2) Contain the chest (like something held in one's mouth) and draw up the back. (*Han Xiong Ba Bei*)

This is to some degree a function of the "Kidney Breathing" (deep abdominal breathing) that is essential to the practice of Nei Gong. When the heart and chest are relatively empty, the spirit is calm and stable. When the lower abdomen is full qi is stored and *Jing* is replenished. When the spirit is calm and stable and the lower abdomen is full, there is stillness inside even as the body moves and changes.

The Nei Gong Triad

In internal martial arts and internal exercises, one needs to engage with the following triad:

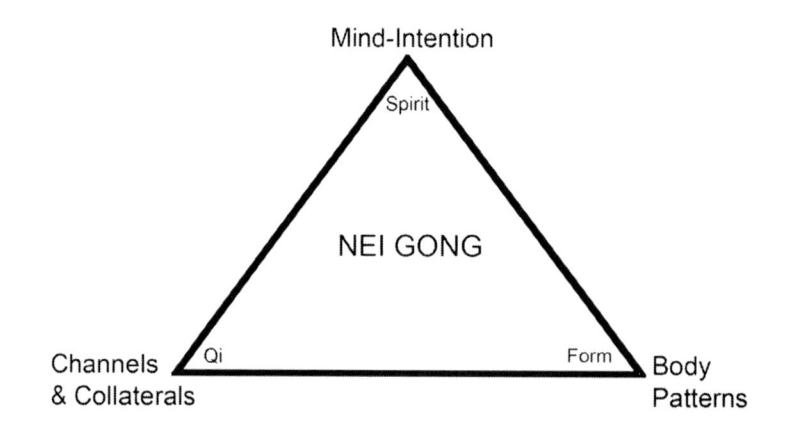

```
                    Mind-Intention
                         /\
                        /Spirit\
                       /        \
                      /          \
                     /  NEI GONG  \
                    /              \
                   /                \
                  /_____\
            Channels  Qi         Form  Body
            & Collaterals              Patterns
```

Teachers of *Nei Gong* and the internal martial arts often say that to really understand these practices, to understand qi and to understand Kan-

28

Water and Li–Fire, one has to understand Chinese medicine. Further, they emphasize three key points that are critical to learning Nei Gong and internal martial arts correctly.

1. It is necessary to have a thorough understanding of the Jing-Luo (meridians) in order to practice Nei Gong correctly
2. It is necessary to have a thorough understanding of the postures and forms, the internal and external body alignments and the methods of moving and changing between the postures and forms.
3. The mind must be tranquil and calm. The mind-intention (Yi) must permeate all postures and movements.

In training and application, these three elements - the three points of the triangle above - operate as an organic and indivisible whole. Interestingly, these same three points are echoed repeatedly in passages from Nei Gong Zhen Chuan (Authentic Classic of Nei Gong):

1. Real knowledge of Nei Gong requires a thorough understanding of the vessels and collaterals.[19]

2. Once the vessels and collaterals are understood you must observe the patterns. After one is familiar with the channels and collaterals it is necessary to understand that there are certain patterns that pertain to the whole body. If the patterns are not understood, all discussion of the channels and collaterals is empty talk.[20]

---

[19] *Nei Gong: The Authentic Classic – A Translation of the Nei Gong Zhen Chuan,* translated by Tom Bisio, Huang Guo-Qi and Joshua Paynter. Outskirts Press Inc, 2011, p. 3.
[20] Ibid, p. 7.

3. Once Zhenqi (True Qi) is sufficient in the interior, its external expression will manifest. Although it is hidden inside and unmoving, numinous brilliance is expressed outwardly through the face so that people cannot look at it directly. The qi stirs from the form, while form follows the qi. The mind is the master of the spirit and the spirit is the master of the qi. Therefore, when the Shenqi takes residence, the form will no longer be a burden and one will be like a dragon soaring in the clouds, a bird flying in the emptiness of the sky, coming suddenly and going.[21]

The base of the triangle above consists of the *Jing-Luo* (channels and collaterals – ie: the meridians) and the body patterns or forms. The channels and collaterals are the pathways of the qi. They are like rivers, lakes, canals and irrigation ditches that spread qi, blood and fluids throughout the body. The Ren Mai (Conception Vessel) and Du Mai (Governing Vessel) which run up along the midline of the body (in the front and back respectively) are the most important vessels to cultivate, open and unblock in inner alchemy, internal martial arts and Nei Gong. *In front is the Ren and in Back is the Du. Between these two the qi turns constantly.*[22] Once these vessels open, it is said that "the hundred meridians will open." When the Eight Extraordinary meridians are open and unblocked, one can connect with the primordial consciousness and the authentic self. However, the channels must not be forced open - they will open up gradually through correct application of form, body patterns and the intention.

Qi does not move easily through tense or blocked areas. The body patterns (*Shi*) set up alignments in which the circulation of qi is not only not

---

[21] Ibid, p. 23.
[22] Ibid, p. 3.

blocked, but is actually augmented and amplified. What is meant by body patterns? *Ding Shi* (定式), or "fixed pattern" circle walking, is perhaps **the** key foundational practice in Ba Gua Zhang. *Ding* means "fixed" or "definite," and at the same time it conveys a sense of calm stability. *Shi* means posture or pattern. Similarly in Xing Yi Quan, San Ti Shi (the "three body posture") is the key Nei Gong practice, which forms the foundation from which all the other movements and techniques manifest. San Ti Shi and Ding Shi are patterns of interconnected and interacting body alignments, akin to the warp and weave of a rug rather than mere external postures. The "pattern" in the context of the practice Xing Yi, Ba Gua and Nei Gong include an interweaving of the body alignments, the intention, qi and *Jin* (劲) – vigor, power, strength.

The opening of the meridians in conjunction with the body patterns not only calms and stabilizes the spirit thereby transforming consciousness, but can only take place when the spirit, in turn, is calm and stable. Therefore, each element of this triad simultaneously acts on and is acted upon, by the other two elements. In this way, internal training is an organic inter-connected, living whole. Understanding in one area of training necessarily facilitates understanding in every other area.

Opening the Meridians

Opening the meridians means to unblock them so that there is an unobstructed flow of vital energy through these pathways. Unblocking and opening the meridians in turn opens the body and mind to the universe around us so that we can sense the health and vitality of our own body in relation to the natural forces that act upon us at every moment. Jonathan Snowiss, a teacher of internal Chinese arts, uses the analogy of a ventilation system. The meridians are like air ducts and the acu-points are like vents on those ducts. If the ducts and vents are closed, the system becomes clogged and the circulation of air is impeded. If they are open, air flows freely and stale air and pathogens can be flushed out and replaced by clean air.[23]

The Du and Ren Channels which run up and down the centerline of the body are the master meridians in the sense that when they open, the other meridians can also open. These two channels form an integrated circuit that is sometimes referred to as the "central channel." It is said that when one meridian opens (the central channel), the hundred meridians can open. So by opening the Ren and Du we facilitate the opening of all the other meridians.

---

[23] *Wei Tuo Qi Gong – Climbing the Mountain: The Essence of Qi Gong and Martial Arts,* by Jonathan Snowiss. Xlibris, 2010, pp.94-5.

Chapter 3
Jing Luo: The Meridian System

Meridians

The Ancient Chinese thought of acu-points as the *microscopic equivalents of the stars in the heavens*.[24] They are not scattered randomly, but are tied together creating patterns similar to small clusters of stars and constellations. This network acts primarily to circulate the qi (vital force).[25] Although meridians and acu-points were thought of as the human embodiments of stars and constellations, the more classic and utilitarian analogy was the similarity of meridians to natural and man-made waterways – rivers, lakes, tributaries, canals, reservoirs and irrigation ditches. In the *Ling Shu*, the twelve meridians are compared to the 12 important rivers of the Emperor Huang Di's era. This analogy emphasized the close connection and symbiosis of man with the natural world by relating the depth and length of the meridians to the depth and length of a particular waterway, thereby also explaining the varied depth of needling in different meridians.[26]

In the 8th century, Wang Ping commented that: *the tracts and the channels (jing-mo) are inside the body and the branches that connect them horizontally are the luo. And the luo again have further branches which are called sun.*[27] The *sun* are smaller bifurcating branches that form a capillary-like network. The term *jing* refers to the warp threads in a piece of fabric and has the meaning to go through, lead, transmit or to direct. *Mai* (or *Mo*)

---

[24] *Celestial Lancets: A History and Rationale of Acupuncture and Moxa*, by Lu Gwei-Djen and Joseph Needham. First published by Cambridge University Press in 1980. Routledge Curzon reprint in 2002, p. 15.
[25] Ibid.
[26] *Huangdii Neijing Ling Shu: Books IV-V with commentary; Vol I*. Nguyen Van Nghi, Tran Viet Dzung, Christine Recours Nguyen. Sugar Grove, NC: Jung Tao Productions 1995 – English Edition 2006, p.283.
[27] Ibid. p. 18.

means "to pulsate." Therefore *jing mai* or *jing mo*, specifically refers to the pulsating vessels within the body that carry blood and vital force. The ancient concept of the *jing mai* clearly apprehended the structures that we associate with modern anatomy and physiology:

- The Blood Vessels (*Xue Mai*)
- The Brain (*Nao*) and Central Nervous System
- The Spinal Cord (*Sui*) and Spinal Nerves
- The Peripheral Nerves and other Nervous System Pathways
- The Tendons and Ligaments (*Jin*) and Muscles (*Ji Rou*) as they are delineated in the Muscle Channels [28] or "Tendino-Muscular Meridians" (TMM)

Luo means "net" or "network," while *jing mai* refers to the main channels and vessels (which primarily run longitudinally). *Luo* refers to the many branches that emanate from these vessels, subdividing and spreading in every direction like the mesh of a net, or like the branches of a tree. Although this all sounds very specific, in practice Chinese medicine employs the terms *mai, jing mai,* and *jing luo* fairly interchangeably. *Mai* can indicate the pulse, in the sense of the palpable rhythmic movement of blood and other substances within the vessels, but *mai* can also indicate the vessels themselves – the veins, arteries and other vessels that form the network that distributes the yin and yang energies throughout the body. In some texts, the *jing luo* are said to carry blood and fluids because the yin and yang energies carried by these vessels include blood, fluids and qi.

The *jing luo* (channels and collaterals) have today largely been replaced by the more modern, yet confusing term, "meridians." When

---

[28] *Anatomical Roots of Chinese Medicine and Acupuncture* by Claus C. Schnorrenberger (After a lecture presented to the British Medical Acupuncture Society, University of Warwick, England, BMAS Spring Meeting 2006.

talking about the *jing luo* or the meridians, it is important to keep in mind that these channels and collaterals are not discrete "energy lines" in the body, but pathways that are congruent with anatomical structures and largely follow and intersect with the circulatory system and its net of capillaries which distribute, blood, fluid, oxygen and nutrients all over the body. In the words of senior acupuncturist, Dr. Wang Ju-Yi:

> *Narrowly speaking, one might say that the channels are "spaces" (jian xi) in the body. In a larger sense, the concept of channel refers not only to the spaces, but to everything wrapped within them. In this definition, the concept broadens to include not only the spaces within the connective tissues, but also the structures (and fluids) held and brought together by these connective tissues. A channel is then like a river in that it includes the riverbanks and also the complexity of life within the water itself held by those banks. In the body, the channels are the groupings of connective tissue, that bring together the blood vessels, bones, lymphatic vessels, nerves, tissues and interstitial fluids within their purview.*[29]

Acu-Points

There are said to be 365 acu-points in the body, a symbolic correlation of the number of degrees in the movements of the heavens (the days of the year), representing another macrocosm-microcosm between heaven and earth and human beings.[30] Acu-points are locations on the body where the movement and distribution of the yin and yang energies

---

[29] *Applied Channel Theory in Chinese Medicine: Wang Ju-Yi's Lectures on Channel Therapeutics* by Wang Ju-Yi and Jason Robertson Seattle: Eastland Press, 2008, p. 13.

[30] *Celestial Lancets: A History and Rationale of Acupuncture and Moxa*, by Lu Gwei-Djen and Joseph Needham. First published by Cambridge University Press in 1980. Routledge Curzon reprint in 2002, p. 15.

circulating in the *jing luo* can be modulated. Points are traditionally described by the character 穴 (*Xue*), meaning "cave" or "hole". Acu-points are sometimes referred to as *Qi Xue* or "qi holes", implying a movement that goes both in and out and follows the channels. They are sometimes defined as pores or interstices in the flesh through which qi and pathogens (evil qi or malign qi) can pass.[31] Many acupuncture points are located along the pathways of the channels and collaterals and are then either referred to by name or by their order of appearance on the channel. For example, *He Gu* ("Valley Meeting"), located on the hand in the web between the thumb and forefinger, is also the fourth point on the Large Intestine Meridian and is therefore also known as "Large Intestine Four" or "LI4". There are also numerous "extra points" not associated with a particular meridian. From an anatomical standpoint, acu-points tend to be located at the spot where peripheral nerves enter a muscle, the midpoint of the muscle, or where the muscle joins with the bone.

The Meridian System

There are 12 Main Channels (*Jing Zheng*) in the body. These are associated with and have direct connections to internal organs like the heart, kidney, gallbladder, stomach etc. These meridians have pathways that connect superficial structures like the sense organs to the body's deeper structures such as the brain and the internal organs. They supply nutrition, fluids and blood to these areas.

The 12 Sinew Channels (*Jing Jin*) are also referred to as the Muscle Channels or Tendino-Muscular Meridians. They form a capillary-like net that spreads through the muscles and tendons, bringing qi and blood to

---

[31] Ibid, p. 14.

these structures. These channels are essentially collaterals of the main meridians that are more superficial in depth. They are indivisible from the bands of muscle, tendon and fascia that form the longitudinal striations that run up and down along the surface of the body. Yang defensive energy flows in these vessels which also connect to the skin and flesh and control the opening and closing of the pores and the venting of heat through the sweat. These channels will not be discussed independently from the main meridians, because in Ba Gua Circle Walking Nei Gong, both the Sinew Channels and the Twelve Main Channels are automatically stimulated through the physical postures and movements.

The Eight Extraordinary Meridians are also known as the "Eight Extra Meridians", the "Curious Vessels" and in Daoist meditation and inner alchemy as the "Eight Psychic Channels". These channels integrate and inter-connect the main channel system and originate at a more primal level than the main meridians. Many acupuncturists speculate that these channels are activated during the embryonic phase of fetal development, well before the main meridians are formed. Therefore, they may serve as a kind of matrix, present from the moment of conception, which is the source of energetic functioning and cellular division and differentiation.[32]

Although acupuncture theory delineates a number of other collateral vessels which are used in medical treatments, specific knowledge of these vessels is much less important in the practice of Ba Gua Nei Gong. Therefore, they will not be discussed here.

---

[32] *Atlas of Acupuncture* by Claudia Focks. Churchill Livingstone (Elsevier Limited), 2008, p. 25)

Yin and Yang Channels

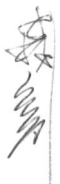

The Twelve main meridians are divided into six yin and yang pairs. The yang meridians - Taiyang, Shaoyang and Yangming - are on the back and the sides of the body, while the yin meridians - Taiyin, Shaoyin and Jueyin – are on the front of the body and inside of the arms and legs. If the sun were behind us and we stood with our palms facing forward, or if we were on all fours like an animal crouching on the ground, the yang surface would roughly be the areas the sun hit directly while the yin areas would be shaded.

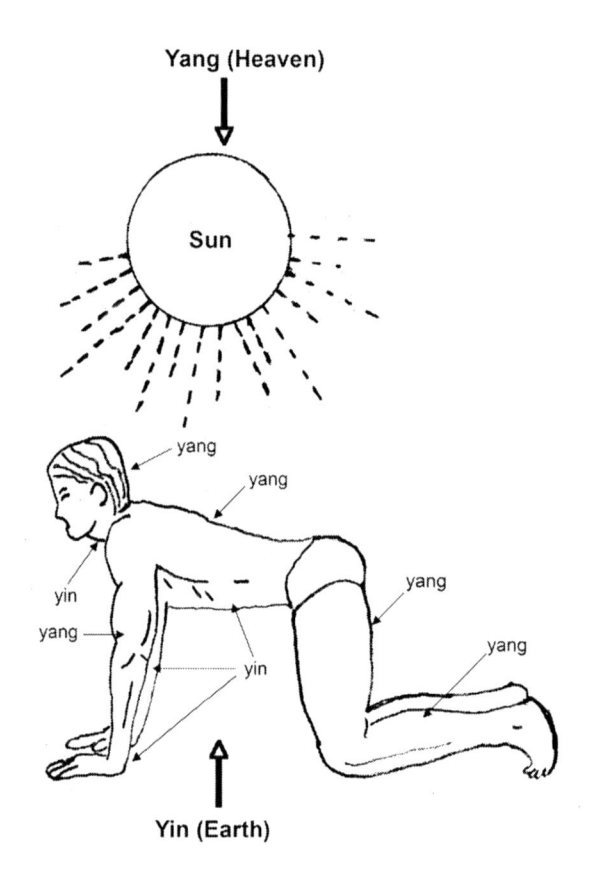

The Channels and Collaterals (*Jing –Luo*/Meridians)

Twelve Main Channels (*Jing Zheng*)

These 12 principle meridians are divided into 6 yin/yang pairings, which aid us in understanding their interconnections and functioning. The pairings are as follows:

Yang Channels

Taiyang
1. Small Intestine Channel of Hand Taiyang
2. Bladder Channel of Foot Taiyang

Shaoyang
3. Triple Heater Channel of Hand Shaoyang
4. Gallbladder Channel of Foot Shaoyang

Yangming
5. Large Intestine Channel of Hand Yangming
6. Stomach Channel of Foot Yangming

Yin Channels

Taiyin
7. Lung Channel of Hand Taiyin
8. Spleen Channel of Foot Taiyin

Shaoyin
9. Heart Channel of Hand Shaoyin
10. Kidney Channel of Foot Shaoyin

Jueyin
11. Pericardium Channel of Hand Jueyin
12. Liver Channel of Foot Jueyin

Twelve Sinew Channels (*Jing Jin*)

These channels are divided similarly to the primary meridians and are interlinked with them:

1. Sinew Channel of Hand Taiyang
2. Sinew Channel of Foot Taiyang
3. Sinew Channel of Hand Shaoyang
4. Sinew Channel of Foot Shaoyang
5. Sinew Channel of Hand Yangming
6. Sinew Channel of Foot Yangming
7. Sinew Channel of Hand Taiyin
8. Sinew Channel of Foot Taiyin
9. Sinew Channel of Hand Shaoyin
10. Sinew Channel of Foot Shaoyin
11. Sinew Channel of Hand Jueyin
12. Sinew Channel of Foot Jueyin

Eight Extraordinary Meridians (*Qi Jing Ba Mai*)

1. Du Mai (Governing Vessel)
2. Ren Mai (Conception Vessel)
3. Chong Mai (Thrusting Vessel)
4. Dai Mai (Belt Vessel)
5. Yang Qiao Mai (Yang Heel Vessel)
6. Yin Qiao Mai (Yin Heel Vessel)
7. Yang Wei Mai (Yang Linking Vessel)
8. Yin Wei Mai (Yin Linking Vessel)

The Meridians and The Fascia

Fascia is fibrous connective tissue that permeates the entire body, binding together and wrapping virtually every structure in the body including the organs, muscles, nerves and blood vessels. *Like ligaments, aponeuroses, and tendons, fasciae are dense regular connective tissues. containing closely packed bundles of collagen fibers oriented in a wavy pattern parallel to the direction of pull. Fasciae are consequently flexible structures able to resist great unidirectional tension forces until the wavy pattern of fibers has been straightened out by the pulling force. These collagen fibers are produced by the fibroblasts located within the fascia.*[33]

The oldest medical manuscripts in China were found in Changsha, in the Mawangdui tombs from the early Han dynasty (2nd century BC). Some of these manuscripts contain longevity techniques and exercises that were used as a means of preventing disease and attaining long life. Many of these exercises depict various kinds of medical exercise, including stretching movements that relieve or "pull" pain from various areas in the body. Some movements depict ways of modifying or balancing yin and yang, while others are described as enhancing qi flow in the eight extraordinary channels.[34]

Donald Harper suggests that these early medical manuscripts combined ideas about muscles and blood vessels leading to what today we call channels and collaterals or meridians.[35] In practice the channels and collaterals interpenetrate with the muscles, fascia, tendons, bone and the internal organs in an interconnected network. The ancient *Dao Yin* exercises

---

[33] http://en.wikipedia.org/wiki/Fascia
[34] *Chinese Healing Exercises* by Livia Kohn, Honolulu: University of Hawai'i Press, 2008, p.43.
[35] *Early Chinese Medical Literature: The Mawangdui Manuscripts*, Translation and Study by Donald Harper. London and New York: Kegan Paul International, 1998, p. 83.

apparently used massage-like movements and stretches to lead, guide and tug the qi in specific ways. Today, Nei Gong practitioners use posture, movement and the breath to contract, relax and align and re-orient the fascia, muscles and tendons, ligaments and bones. These actions in turn stretch, and open and close the meridians, while simultaneously expanding and contracting the cavities that contain the internal organs.

Many modern practitioners of Traditional Chinese medicine feel that the fascial network that binds all of these structures together has significant congruence with the ancient concepts of the channels and collaterals. Nei Gong and Qi Gong traditions employ movement in coordination with mind-intention in order to modify the functional activities (the "qi-dynamic") that Chinese medicine attributes to the internal organs. These physiological effects can be understood to operate to some degree by modification of the flow of qi and fluids through the fascia and the jing luo system.

In Osteopathic medicine, the movement of interstitial fluid through the body is felt to precede the development of the cardio-vascular system in embryonic development. This fluid motion, which moves rhythmically through the body, is like a tide that brings nutrients to cells and carries away cellular wastes. W. G. Sutherland, famous for his teachings in Cranial Osteopathy, referred to this motion as the "Tide of Life."[36]

> *In other words, the capillary beds are hooked together into one big grid. Closer observation of this same histological section reveals that the individual cells are organized into a matrix, which creates channels by which the nutrient-rich fluids of the body travel to supply all the cells equally, even those farthest from the source. The primary*

---

[36] *Ligamentous Articular Strain: Osteopathic Manipulative Techniques for the Body,* by Conrad A. Speece, D.O. and William Thomas Crow, D.O., Seattle: Eastland Press, 2001, p. 27.

> *respiratory mechanism pushes fluids into these matrices, creating fluid waves within the body. It is this hydrodynamic fluctuation that nourishes every cell.*[37]

Helene Langevin, Ph.D., a scientist working at the University of Vermont, and her colleagues have done research that suggests an overlap between the fascia and the channels and collaterals. They have effectively demonstrated that acu-points, and many of the effects of acupuncture, seem to relate to the fact that most of these acu-points lie directly over areas where there is a fascial cleavage – ie: where sheets of fascia diverge to separate, surround and support different muscle bundles.[38] The meridians may be, at least in part, fascial pathways. This is not too surprising, since we know the fascial network represents a unified continuum, from the internal cranial reciprocal tension membranes to the plantar fascia of the feet.[39] This fascial network was clearly understood by traditional Chinese physicians who referenced this network as the Sinew Channels or Tendino-Muscular Meridians. Langevin and others speculate that the connective tissue network is a sophisticated communication system of yet unknown potential:

> *'Loose' connective tissue forms a network extending throughout the body including subcutaneous and interstitial connective tissues. The existence of a cellular network of fibroblasts within loose connective tissue may have considerable significance as it may support yet unknown body-wide cellular signaling systems. ...Our findings indicate that soft tissue fibroblasts form an extensively interconnected*

---

[37] Ibid.
[38] *Relationship of Acupuncture Points and Meridians to Connective Tissue Planes,* by Helene M. Langevin and Jason A. Yandow. The Anatomical Record (New Aant.) 269:257–265, 2002.
[39] The *Amazing Fascial Web, Part I,* By Leon Chaitow, ND, DO. *Massage Today* May, 2005, Vol. 05, Issue 05.

cellular network, suggesting they may have important, and so far unsuspected integrative functions at the level of the whole body.[40]

---
[40] Ibid.

Chapter 4
Ding Shi Ba Gua Nei Gong: Basic Alignments and Body Patterns

Ding Shi and Circle Walking

Ding Shi (定 式) or Fixed Pattern circle walking is perhaps **the** key foundational practice in Ba Gua Zhang. **Ding** means "fixed" or "definite," and at the same time it conveys a sense of calm stability. **Shi** means posture or pattern. Thinking of the Eight Ding Shi as patterns of interconnected and interacting body alignments is more useful than thinking of them as external postures. Understanding the Ding Shi as "body patterns" will aid you in performing Ding Shi Ba Gua correctly and help you to understand its role as the primary Ba Gua Nei Gong exercise. The "Pattern," in the context of Ba Gua and Nei Gong, includes an interweaving of the body alignments, the intention, the qi and the *jin* 劲 (vigor, power, strength).

Holding fixed postures while walking in a circle builds strength and develops unified whole-body power. Before changing from one posture or pattern to another, one must first learn to relax the body so that it is comfortable in the fixed pattern. Once you can hold the pattern and walk for period of time without discomfort, then you can begin to focus more on changing from one posture to another.

In practicing the Ding Shi we walk around a circle using the "mud wading step" (*Tang Ni Bu*). Although the image is one of lifting and setting down the foot like one is wading through mud, the purpose of this "mud stepping" is to walk in a flowing and rooted way. The steps curve and the body turns, creating a dynamic driving force that is both relaxed and stable. The foot lifts and treads down with the sole of the foot parallel to the floor. Training the step in this way not only creates stability and mobility, but also links the power of the legs with the turning of the waist so that the legs, the low back and the waist act as a single unit. Mud stepping on a circle while holding the Ding Shi postures produces a natural winding power which is stored and released continuously with each step.

The mud step allows you to change the direction of the step at the last possible minute. This is also easier if the step is curved rather than straight. The curved step has many functions.

In Nei Gong:

1. The curved step combined with the turning of the back and waist and the folding of the *kua*[41] creates a series of spiral forces that run through the fascia from the sole of the foot through the entire body, creating a unified structure that is akin to a twisted rope. These spiral forces activate and invigorate the qi.

2. The action of lifting and setting down the foot activates two important acu-points: *Mingmen* (DU 4), which lies just in front of the spine in the middle of the lower back; and *Yong Quan* (KID 1), a point on the sole of the foot. These two points in turn activate the kidney meridian and the Ren and Du channels so that the primal energies of the body and their pathways - the Eight Extraordinary Vessels - are stimulated and opened.

3. The rotation of the body combined with walking in a circle moves qi, blood and fluids through the entire *jing-luo* system. This clears and opens the channels and collaterals and stimulates the qi mechanism of the body. This in turn activates the body's defensive energies helping it to dispel pathogens and improve functioning of the internal organs, thereby stimulating circulation, digestion, and elimination.

---

[41] "kua" refers to the inguinal area in the front of the pelvis, including both the internal and external structures of the inguinal area and the movement of qi and fluids through that area.

This clearing and opening action helps to unblock the channels and collaterals, preventing stagnation which is considered to be the root of many diseases in Chinese medicine.

4. Rotating and walking harmonizes the body's energies with the cyclical circular movements of the earth, the stars and the planets. This connects us to the natural forces of which we are a part. In turn this connection allows the mind to become quiet and tranquil and the heart becomes calm and relaxed. Then the spirit becomes rooted and serene.

In Martial Applications:

1. The curved step in combination with the turning of the back and waist and the folding of the *kua* allows you to turn the opponent's force so that it is deflected and guided around you, thereby allowing you to move behind him.
2. The curved step creates a deception that we are moving to the side or even retreating when we are actually moving forward.
3. The curved step allows you to cover and control the eight directions by simply walking forward.

The Downward Sinking Palm

In learning to walk the circle you will begin with the Downward Sinking Palm. In each practice session, you will always begin with the Downward Sinking Palm. There are two reasons for this:

1. The Downward Sinking Palm settles the body weight downward into the feet so that the body is rooted and stable.//
2. The Downward Sinking Palm opens the Ren, Du and Chong Vessels – three of the Eight Extraordinary meridians that help connect and regulate all of the other meridians. This will be discussed in detail in subsequent chapters.

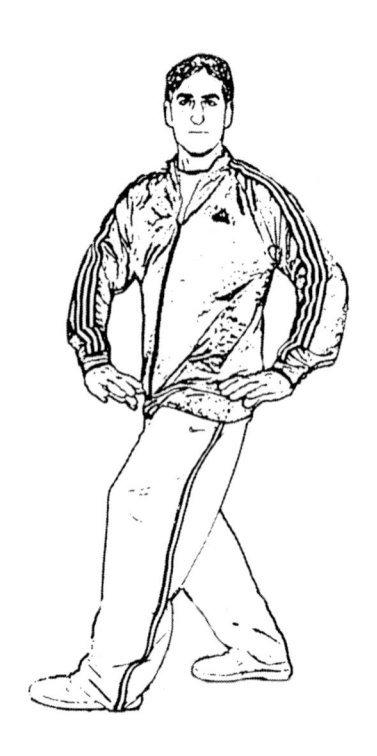

Downward Sinking Palm: Stationary Practice

Stand on the periphery of the circle, facing counterclockwise. With the feet close together, bend the knees slightly and press downward until the palms are below the waist in front of the hips. The palm root sinks down and the fingers of each hand point toward each other. It should feel as though you are pushing a ball down gently into the water. The palms are in front of each hip. They should sink down, but simultaneously feel like they are being pushed upward. The palms feel like they are pulling apart and rotating inward while they also feel as though they are rotating inward and drawing toward each other. The upper body lifts upward and the lower body sinks downward. Check all the body alignments discussed below.

Now step the left foot out and let the right kua[42] fold so that the body turns leftward toward the inside of the circle. As you turn, make sure that the shoulders and palms stay level. The turning and folding of the kua "screws" the right leg into the ground so that you are rooted on the right leg. Again check all the body alignments discussed below. Then try this facing clockwise on the circle. Step the right foot out and let the left kua fold so that the body turns toward the inside of the circle (toward the right).

Linear Mud Stepping: The Slow Walk

The easiest way to learn mud stepping is to do it very slowly in a straight line with small steps. Later on you will vary the steps and walk on a circle at different speeds. The key is to move slowly, evenly and smoothly. **For now, it should take 1-2 minutes to take a single step.** As you practice mud stepping, use the downward pressing palm and maintain the following alignments and check the detailed discussion of the alignments that follow this section:

- The head erects and lifts upward and the tail sinks downward
- The tongue tip touches the upper palate
- The shoulders are relaxed and sink downward

---

[42] See previous footnote.

- The skeleton feels like it lifts upward while the flesh sinks downward
- The shoulders and hips are level.

The Slow Walk

1. **Start:** With your feet together and the weight evenly distributed between the two feet, bend your knees slightly and fold the *kua* as the arms assume the position of the downward sinking palm. (Fig. 1)

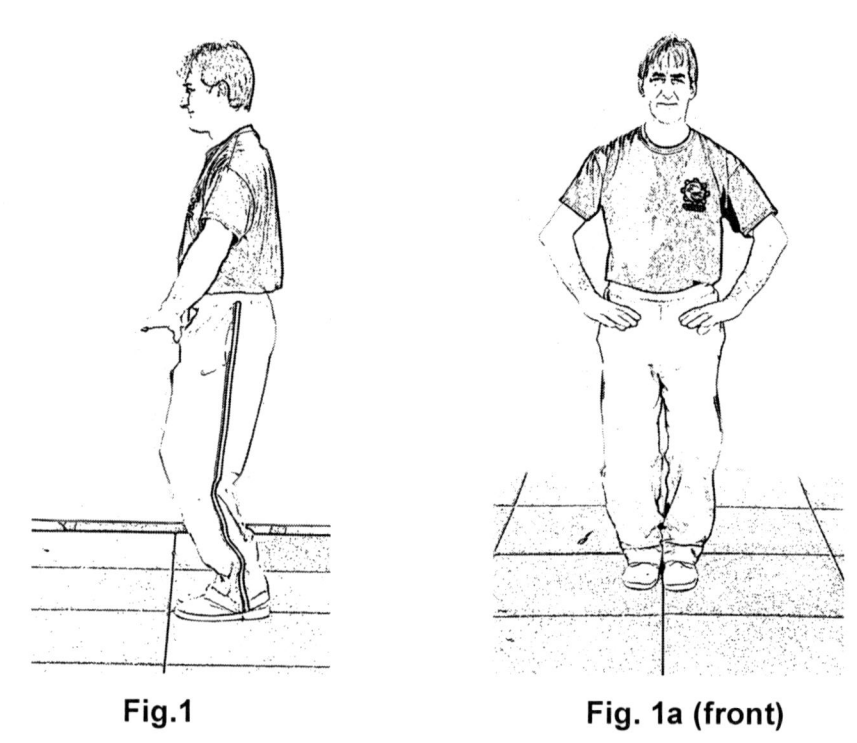

Fig.1 **Fig. 1a (front)**

2. Slowly lift the left foot off the floor. The whole sole lifts at the same time.
3. Step the left foot out a few inches. As it steps, the foot is just off the floor. As it moves forward, the foot should feel as though you are pushing a brick forward with the toes. (Fig. 2)
4. The step is slow and even. Pause for a moment with the foot just off the floor before it sets down on the floor with no weight. (Fig. 3)

Fig. 2   **Fig. 3**

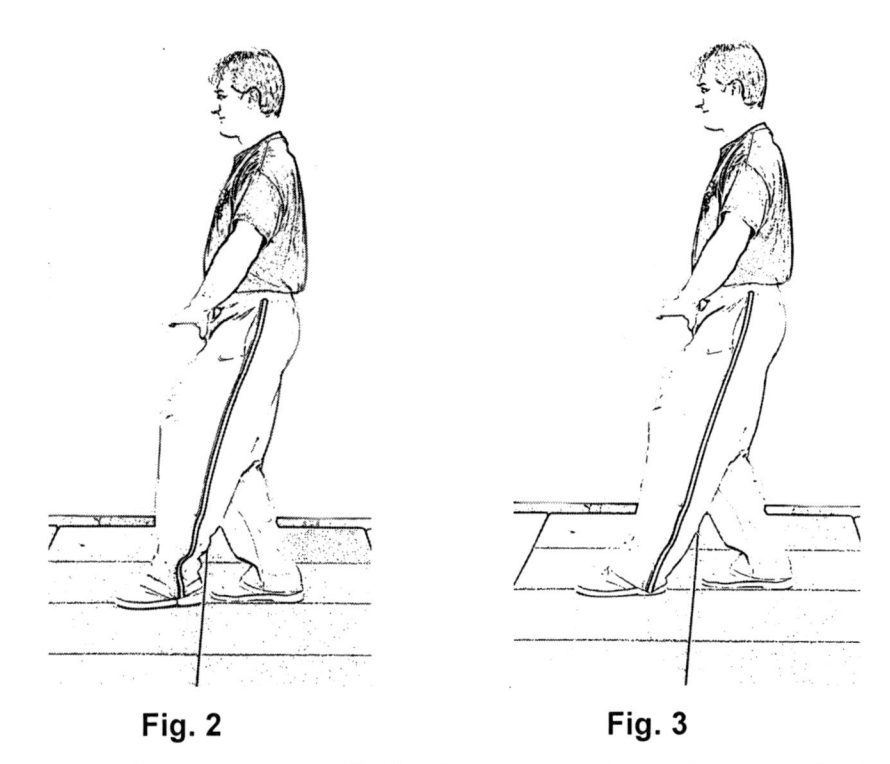

5. **Now the exercise really begins:** As weight settles onto the foot, feel the whole foot on the floor. Let the foot mold to the floor. The *Yong Quan* (KID 1) on the bottom of the foot will naturally hollow as weight is transferred. Keep the hip, knee and foot in a line as much as possible and keep the hips level as the weight transfers (Fig 4).

6. Transfer weight onto the left foot, keeping the head erect and tail sinking. This should occur very slowly. Once the weight is fully on the left foot, the tips of the right toes will feel like they want to come off the floor. Lift the toes and then lift the arch of the foot (Fig.5).

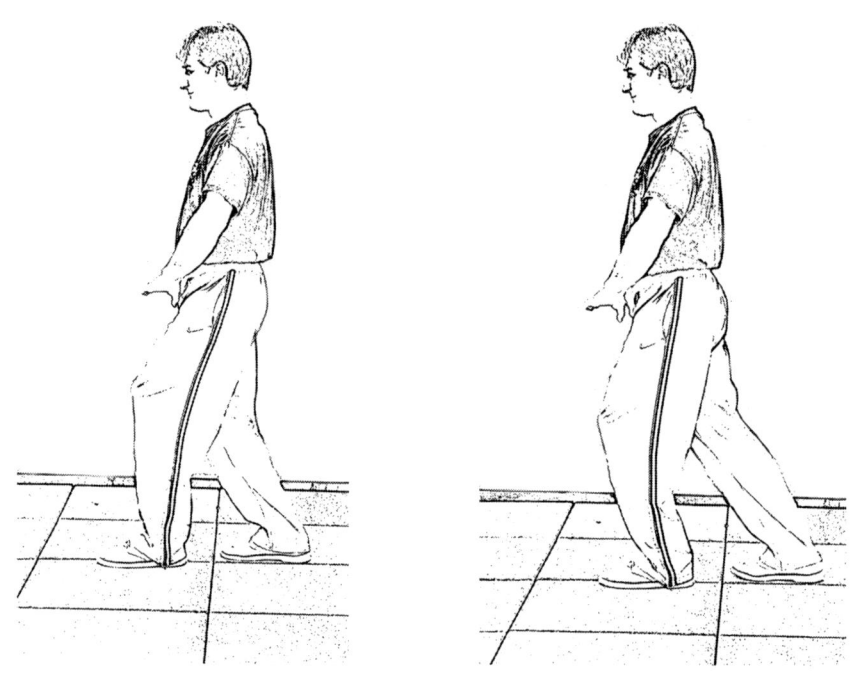

Fig 4.   **Fig. 5**

7. As the heel begins to lift, the sole of the whole foot leaves the floor at once. Step the right foot slowly forward so that it almost brushes the ground as it moves. As it moves forward, the foot should feel as though you are pushing a brick forward with the toes (Figs. 6-7).

8. The step is slow. It should take about one-and-a-half to two minutes for the right foot to lift and pass the right leg to step several inches in front of the left foot. The feet move on either side of an imaginary line on the floor. As the foot comes to the end of the step, there is a slight pause at this point with the sole of the right foot parallel to the floor (Figs. 8-9).

Fig. 6

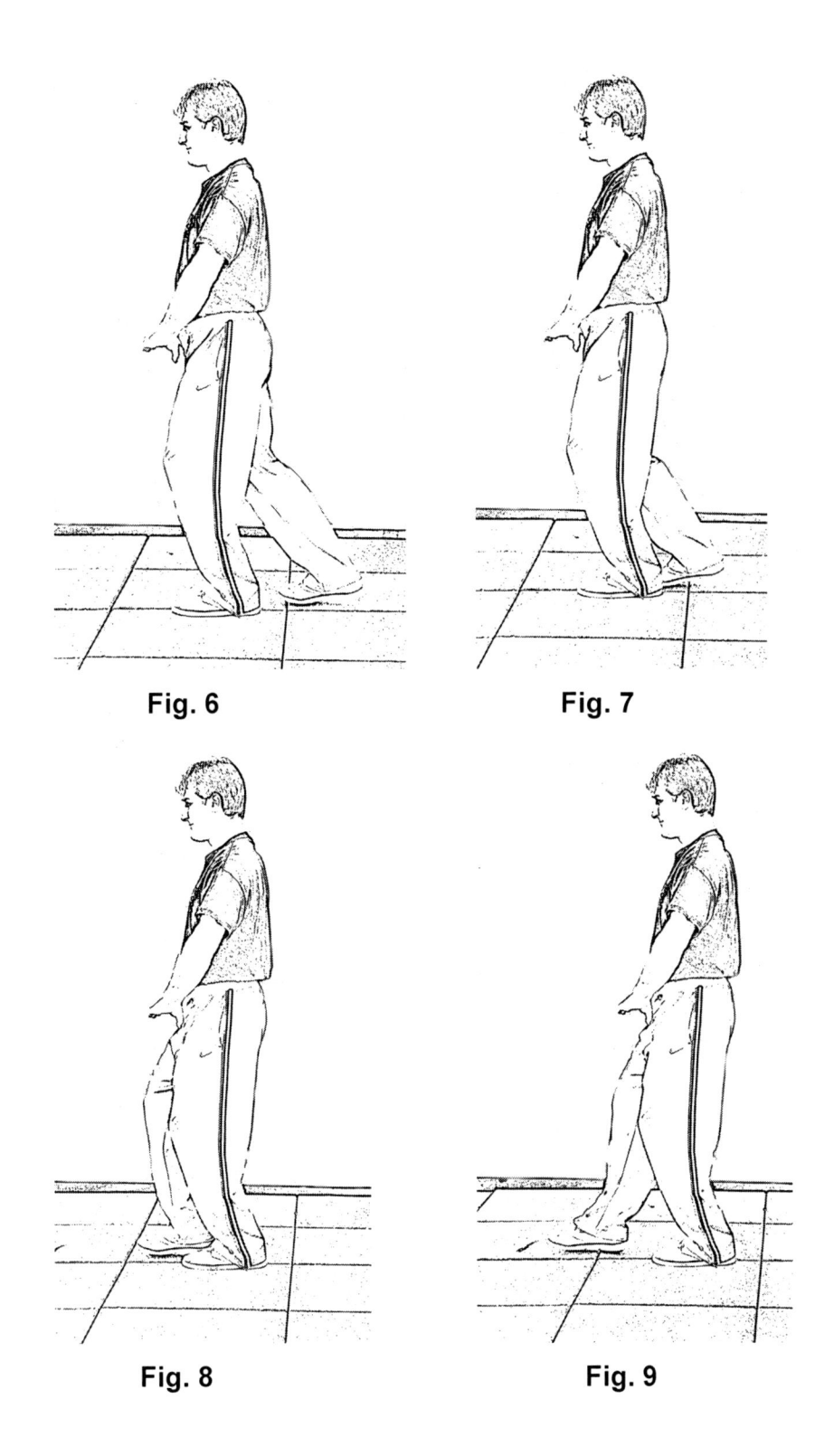

Fig. 7

Fig. 8

Fig. 9

9. Then the foot settles on the floor with no weight (Fig.10).

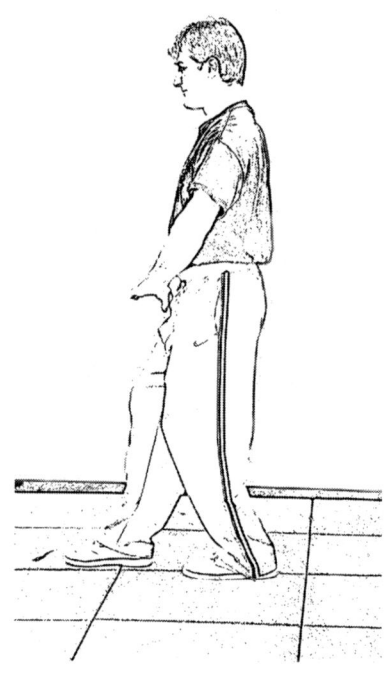

Fig. 10

10. Repeat steps 3-10 with the left foot stepping.
11. Take 3-5 steps per leg in a practice session. This can be done twice a day. Remember to take 1-2 minutes to make a single step.

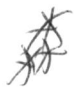

As you practice the Slow Walk, observe internally what is happening as you practice stepping. Attend to the alignment, the breath and the movements. This is an opportunity to observe the precise mechanics of the step and the interplay of the joints, muscles, bones and tendons as you move through the step. At this moment, the slower the step, the better. Later it will be useful to increase the speed of the step.

Mud stepping balances the strength of the muscles in the front, back, inside and outside of the leg. It also connects the power of the legs to the waist, back and upper torso so that power flows continuously from the legs as you move and is transferred seamlessly to the upper body and arms.

Important Considerations:

- Move slowly and evenly throughout the exercise. There is no acceleration or deceleration, but a constant forward movement of the foot.
- The ASIS (the Superior Anterior Iliac Spine (the bump on the front of the hipbone), the knee and the LIV 3 (*Tai Chong*) acu-point remain in a line throughout. *Tai Chong* is in the hollow between the big toe and 2nd toe.
- Resist the tendency to let the hip slide sideways as the weight shifts. Instead hold the hips level.
- Keep breathing. Do not hold the breath. Use Kidney Breathing (see chapter 6).
- Relax. If your knee or ankle are wobbling, focus on the synergistic body alignments rather than the joint that is having difficulty. By focusing on the interconnection of **all** the alignments it will be easier to stabilize a particular joint.

If you have never practiced mud-stepping or circle walking before, spend two or three weeks practicing this exercise using the Downward Sinking Palm twice a day before trying to walk on the circle.

General Body Alignments in Walking the Circle

Both the general body alignments in walking the circle and the specific body alignments of each fixed posture combine to the create the "pattern" (Shi) of the posture. Below is a list of the general alignments that are the same for all eight Ding Shi patterns. Other alignments specific to the individual Ding Shi postures will be discussed in Chapter Five. The alignments work synergistically with each other – that is, each one aids the others, creating a network of interlinked forces and intentions. Focusing too much on one alignment usually creates an imbalanced structure or pattern.

1. Straighten the Neck Slightly and Uplift the Head

The top of the head feels as though it is suspended from the vertex. This, combined with a slight withdrawing of the chin, straightens the neck slightly. This action should be relaxed and unforced, a function of the intention rather than the muscles.

2. Hold and "Lift" the Perineum While Dropping the Tailbone

The buttocks do not stick out and are said to be "smooth" - not sticking out even a little. This is a function of the lower back and tail sinking down while the upper back and neck lift upward (see #1 above). When the neck is straightened and the head uplifted with the tail sinking down, it is easy to feel as though the perineum and anus lift and hold upward. This again is a function of the intention rather than the muscles – i.e. the anus is not forcibly contracted but has a sensation of uplifting. This prevents qi that is accumulating in *Dantian* from leaking out. The perineum or anus are sometimes referred to as the "grain duct." Lifting and upholding the anus allows qi to raise to the Dantian and then from the Dantian to the vertex so

56

that qi can circulate qi freely. This is sometimes referred to as: *"gather the anus and uphold the qi internally."*

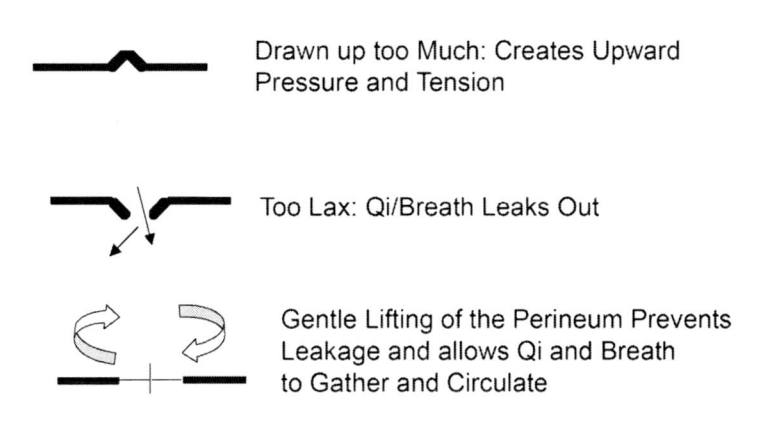

Drawn up too Much: Creates Upward Pressure and Tension

Too Lax: Qi/Breath Leaks Out

Gentle Lifting of the Perineum Prevents Leakage and allows Qi and Breath to Gather and Circulate

The Perineum is Like a Valve

3. Slacken (Song) the Shoulders and Sink the Elbows

The shoulders sink and release downward. The word *Song* is often translated as: to "slacken," "loosen" or "unbind." In walking the circle, it is easy to unintentionally lift one shoulder or the other or to tilt the body so that one shoulder looks higher. Therefore it is important to keep the shoulders level and sinking. Another way to think of this is that loosening the shoulder keeps the chest relaxed and prevents it from sticking out. The elbows also sink downward constantly. This protects the body and aids the shoulders in slackening and loosening. Even when the elbows appear to be raised, they still have a downward sinking orientation.

4. Fingers Separated with the Palm Concave

As the shoulders loosen and the elbows sink, force and energy move out into the hands. The hands curve so that the fingers separate and the palm center is hollow or concave. This occurs naturally as a result of the shoulder and elbow alignments. A good visualization is to feel the hand curve and expand, as though it is a balloon that fills with air, or a limp hose that expands as it fills with water. There are several ways to hold the palm but for now use the "Tile Palm." In the Tile Palm, the thumb stretches toward the pinky rounding the back of the hand like a roof tile. The fore-finger stretches outward and the Tiger's Mouth (Houkou) – the space between the thumb and forefinger - is round and open. The other fingers spread apart in a gentle curve.

5. Touch the Tongue-Tip to the Roof of the Mouth

Just as the head and anus uplift, the tongue also uplifts so that the tip of the tongue touches the roof of the mouth behind the upper teeth. In Daoist meditation this is the "upper magpie gate" which links the Ren and Du Channels above in the mouth. The "lower magpie gate" is created by upholding the anus which links these two channels in the lower body. Once linked and open, they form (along with Chong Mai) the "central channel."

6. Chest Contained and Unimpeded; Abdomen Solid and Full

While the upper back uplifts slightly due to the lifting of the vertex and the straightening of the neck, the chest stays contained and relaxed. The slight rounding of the shoulders that occurs as the shoulders loosen and the elbows sink makes the chest look slightly concave – but again, this is due to the other alignments rather than a collapsing of the chest. The chest is therefore said to be relatively empty and the Dantian relatively full. This is also a result of kidney breathing filling the Dantian. When the abdomen (Dantian) is "full" the body is rooted and powerful and the chest is relaxed, calm and receptive.

7. Sit the Kua and Bend the Knees

The character 胯 (kua) is often mistranslated "hip". It actually refers to the inguinal area in the front of the pelvis, including both the internal and external structures of the inguinal area and the movement of qi and fluids through that area. "Sitting the kua" refers to folding the kua as though sitting down. As you walk the circle, the kua folds and you sit into the legs. The knees bend and weight is transferred into the ground through the soles of the feet. Sinking the tail and smoothing the buttocks (see #2 above) aid the kua in sitting and the knees in bending. Remember, this is balanced by the perineum, the tongue, and the head, neck and upper back uplifting and straightening. The amount of sitting and bending of the knees will depend on the individual. In the beginning, sitting down a little is fine.

8. Mud Wading Step with the Sole of the Foot Empty

In the mud wading step, the foot stays level, meaning that the sole stays parallel to the ground. The foot lifts without showing the heel. For example, if the right foot steps forward as weight transfers to the right foot, the kua sits and the tail sinks, while the upper back and neck lift upward. At a certain point, as most of the weight is on the right foot, you will feel as though the toes of the left foot are starting to lift. The toes lift and then the arch lifts. At that point, lift the whole left foot with the sole parallel to the ground and move it slowly forward with the sole facing the ground. The foot glides just above the ground. It appears to slide on the floor, but does not slide on the floor. When setting the left foot down, the whole foot treads down with the *Yong Quan* ("Bubbling Spring" – KID 1) acu-point hollow. This point is in the hollow in the center of the ball of the foot. Do not tense the foot to make the sole hollow. Rather the foot is like a suction cup that automatically grips the floor. The "hollow" lifting sensation at *Yong Quan* and the suction cup quality come from all the body alignments working synergistically together rather then an active gripping with the foot and leg muscles. The same lifting, gliding and treading action will occur whether the foot on the inside of the circle steps in *Bai Bu* (Swing Step), or whether the foot on the outside of the circle lifts and steps in *Kou Bu* (Hook Step).

9. Tread the Foot, Scissor the Thighs, and Rub the Shins

In walking with the mud step, it feels as though the foot lifts from inside the body rather than from the peripheral leg muscles. This engages the deep torso muscles in moving the leg, including the psoas muscle which connects the femur to the front of the lower lumbar vertebrae. As the leg moves forward, the thighs brush past each other like scissors opening and closing. The shins are said to "grind" or "rub," meaning that the shins pass closely by each other and the leg and foot do not swing too wide. As the sole lifts off the floor and the foot moves forward, it should feel as though you are pushing a brick along the floor with your foot. This "pushing" is slow, even and constant. As soon as the foot sets down, the other foot begins to lift and push.

10. Shoulders Stay Level and the Arms "Swing"

The body and the arms rotate and turn toward the center of the circle, rather than pushing straight ahead. But in turning and rotating, the shoulders must remain level and the body must be comfortable. The turning comes not from twisting the spine, but from folding the kua inward and letting the arms "swing" or turn toward the center of the circle. Ultimately, with practice the turning will emanate from the "Central Channel."

11. Ming Men "Open" and Still

The Ming Men and the central channel are relatively still as the body turns moving around the circle. They are like a hub at the center of a wheel. The sinking of the tail and the lifting of the head and upper back put a gentle traction on the whole spine and "open" Ming Men, while at the same time keeping the spine from kinking and twisting as you turn around the circle. In his *Explanation of the Eight Diagram Palm,* the famous Ba Gua and Xing Yi exponent Jiang Rong Qiao, explained this as follows:

> *Yao like and axle,*
>
> *Hands like Revolving Wheels.*[43]

Remember, although the Ming Men acu-point lies between the second and third lumbar vertebrae, Ming Men itself is located inside the body, in front of the spine. The *yao* (center of the small of the back) is the axis of the movements. When the body turns while walking the circle, the *yao* drives the movements of the arms, turning minutely like the center of the axle. In this sense the center of the *yao*, located at the Ming Men and the central channel is still, like the center of the axle. The arms are like the spokes of a wheel. As the axle turns the spokes also must turn.

The Ming Men is not a single point on the surface of the body, but rather an area that lies inside the body in front of the spine and between the kidneys. Ming Men lies on the central channel and is considered to be directly related or even equivalent to the Dan Tian. Although the acu-point DU 4 is called Ming Men, the area called Ming Men can only be sensed internally – it cannot be located externally.

---

[43] *Ba Gua Zhang*, by Jiang Rong-Qiao, translated by Huang Guo Qi and Tom Bisio.

12. Stand Like a Mountain and Move Like Flowing Water

The purpose of mud stepping and the Ding Shi practice is to develop a "moving root." This means in each step you are stable and rooted to the ground – *"stable as a lofty mountain."* This also means the body stays upright and balanced, without tilting, leaning, or toppling over. At the same time you must also be mobile, able to change direction at will. Although in the beginning you will walk slowly, later the steps must be quick, light and agile. Another traditional way of expressing this dynamic is: *"move like the wind and stand like a nail."*

Training Tip

In beginning, as you walk, go through these alignments like a checklist. This means attending to the whole body at once with an attentive and observant mind. In time, many of the alignments that make up the "body patterns" will fall into place automatically. If you have difficulty with any one part of the body don't focus too much attention on it – **attend to all the alignments and their inherent synergy will correct the problem.**

Chapter 5
Walking the Circle

Kou Bu and Bai Bu: Hooking and Swinging Steps

When walking the circle, the feet make **kou bu** (hook steps) and **bai bu** (swing steps). The outside foot will hook (kou) and the inside foot will walk "straight" along the line that has been set by the hook step. When the outside foot hooks (kou bu) it turns from the kua so that the toes of the inside foot now face the center of the arch of the outside foot. Then the inside foot steps, first going toward the center of the arch of the outside foot, and then "swinging" (bai bu) outward on a curve to follow the line of the outside foot. This is graphically illustrated in the diagram below.

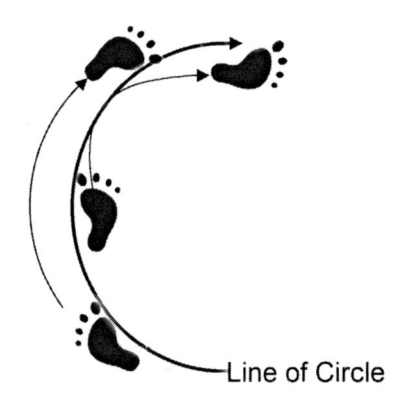

Kou Bu and Bai Bu
Circle Walking

This combination of hooking and swinging - kou and bai – carries you smoothly around the circle. The diagram below is representation of how this would look on circle that takes eight steps to complete.

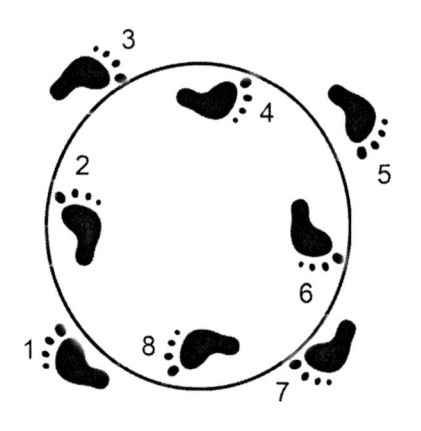

Walking the Circle

In the beginning it is best to use a circle of eight or twelve steps. If it is possible, you can draw a circle on the floor or walk around a post or tree to give you a sense of the center of the circle. Otherwise simply imagine that you are on a circle. The first few times it may be useful to pace out eight natural steps to get a sense of the size of the circle, although ultimately it is through the mud-stepping circle walking practice itself that the correct size will be found.

Start standing on the periphery of the circle, facing counterclockwise. Bend the knees slightly and press downward until the palms are below the waist in front of the hips. The palm root sinks down and the fingers of each hand point toward each other. It should feel as though you are pushing a ball down gently into the water. The palms are in front of each hip. They should sink down, but simultaneously feel like they are being pushed upward. The palms feel like they are pulling apart and rotating outward. At the same time, they feel as though they are rotating inward and drawing toward each other. The upper body lifts upward and the lower body sinks downward.

Kou Bu: Start with the outside step (right). Lift the foot with the sole parallel to the floor and move the foot along the line of the circle, the foot gliding just above the floor. As the foot moves along the periphery of the circle it hooks inward, turning the body. The hook step ends with the center of the inner arch in line with the toes of the left foot. Remember the hooking comes not from the knee, ankle and foot, but from the hip and kua.

Bai Bu: Now move the left foot. Lift the foot with the sole parallel to the floor. The foot glides just above the floor as it first moves directly toward the center of the right foot. Just before the toes of the left foot reach the center of the arch of the right foot, the left foot "swings," arcing to follow the line of the right "hooked" foot. As the foot swings, the body turns with it.

Because the outside foot hooks and the inside foot swings to follow the line of the outside ("hooked") foot, Chinese teachers say that in walking the circle: **the outside foot hooks [Kou Bu] and inside foot walks straight [Bai Bu].**

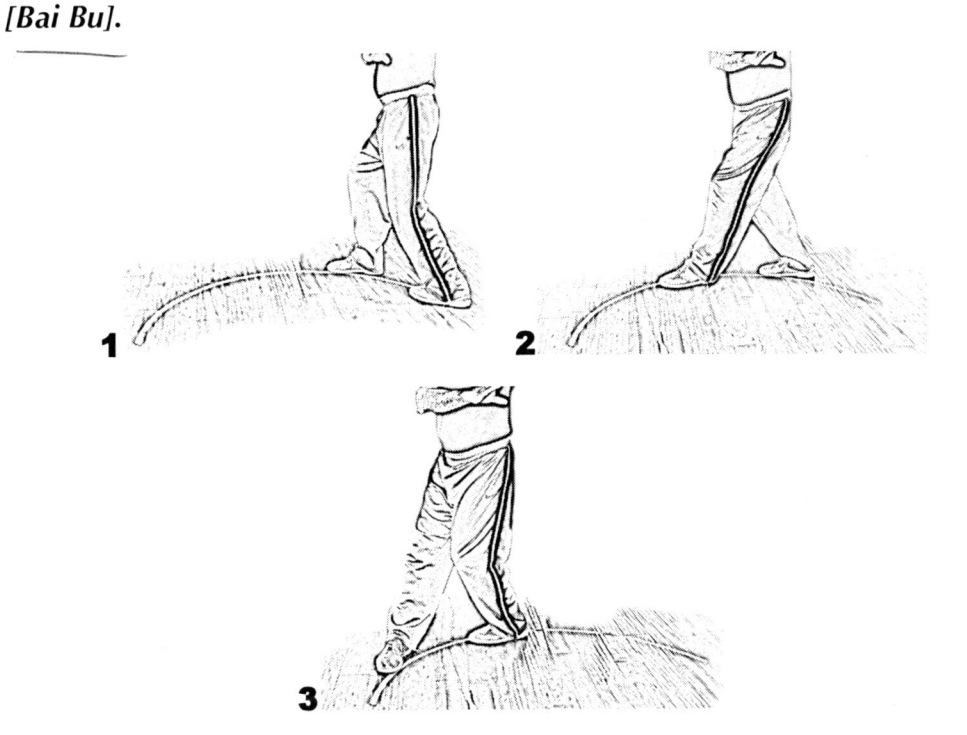

Walking The Circle

Training Tip

In walking the circle, we essentially step from one Yong Quan acu-point to the other with each step. The whole foot is on the floor, but the area around the Yong Quan point makes contact with the floor as the foot lands. Immediately the weight begins to transfer, driving the body forward so the weight does not settle back toward the heel. This creates a constant forward driving action.

The Yong Quan acu-point and the area around it act like a suction cup - the center of the point does not touch the floor but feels like it is sucked upward. This is not a result of contraction of the musculature of the foot and lower leg, but rather the natural result of the other body alignments combining to root the foot while creating a lifting force (ie: The gripping action of the sole of the foot is a result of the upward movement of the head and upper back and the sinking of the tailbone; the lifting of the perineum and the placing of the tongue on the roof of the mouth, etc.).

Walking the Circle in the Downward Sinking Palm Pattern

Start by walking an eight or twelve step circle holding the pattern/posture of the Downward Sinking Palm.

1. Start standing on the periphery of the circle, facing clockwise. Assume pattern/posture of the Downward Sinking Palm:

- Sink the palms downward and as you rotate the arms inward, letting the chest and shoulders round slightly. There is a feeling of space in each armpit.
- The fingertips of both hands point inward to face each other while the thumbs point at the two kua.

- Internally the palms rotate inward and move toward each other while simultaneously there is a feeling of them rotating outward and pulling apart. These two forces balance each other so that the body feels relaxed and supple, yet loaded like a coiled spring.
- It should feel as though you are pushing a ball down gently into the water.
- The sinking of the arms is a function of the sinking of the tailbone and sacrum opposed by the uplifting of the head and upper back. This is aided by sitting the kua and bending the knees so the weight falls through the Yong Quan acu-point – simultaneously there is an internal feeling of straightening through the knees and pushing upward from the soles of the feet. These forces also balance and cancel each other.
- The fingers of each hand are separate and the palm center is hollow. The hands are assume the shape of the "tile palm" (see general body alignment #4 in Chapter 4).

2. Walk clockwise: the left (outside) foot making Kou Bu (hook) steps, while the right makes Bai Bu (swing) steps. As you begin to walk the body will rotate inward so that the palms move toward the center of the circle.

3. Walk for 5 minutes clockwise and then turn. We will start with a four-step turn that helps develop the Kou Bu and Bai Bu steps.

> **Turn Step 1:** Begin to turn by using a left Kou Bu (hook step) with the left foot. Step farther than usual with the left hook step so that as you settle onto the left foot both feet point inward. Chinese teachers often

describe the feet in this position as resembling the shape of the Chinese Character *Ba* (Eight):

八 Eight (*Ba*)

Turn Step 2: Now Bai Bu with the right foot so that you swing the body outward to begin face the outside of the circle.

Turn Step 3: Follow with the left foot making another Kou Bu with the body facing the outside of the circle. The body turns rightward.

Turn Step 4: As the body turns back to the left, move the left foot outward in a swing step stepping along the periphery of the circle. Throughout steps 1-4 use the mud step and maintain the body pattern of the Downward Sinking Palm - lift the foot as though extracting it from thick mud and keep the sole parallel to the floor and just above the floor as you step.

4. Walk Counter-Clockwise For Five minutes: The left foot is now the inside step which will Bai Bu (swing) and the right foot is the outside step which will Kou Bu (hook) as you walk the circle.

Line of Circle
Turn: Step 1

Line of Circle
Turn: Step 2

Line of Circle
Turn: Step 3

Line of Circle
Turn: Step 4

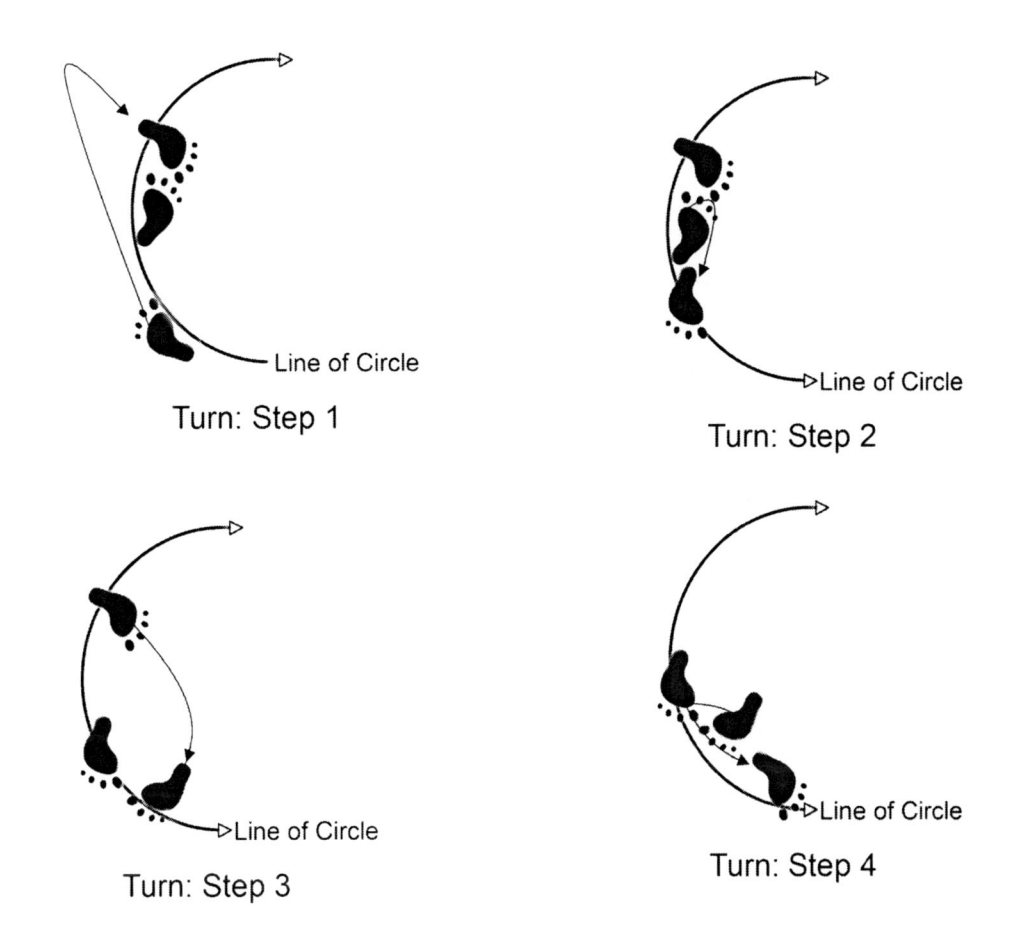

5. End by using Kou Bu to face the center of the circle and raising the arms up with an inhale and then exhale and pressing the palms down to Dantian. Stand still for minute. While the body is externally still, observe the internal movements occurring within the body. The mind observes but is quiet, relaxed and stable.

1　　　　　　　　　　　　　　**2**

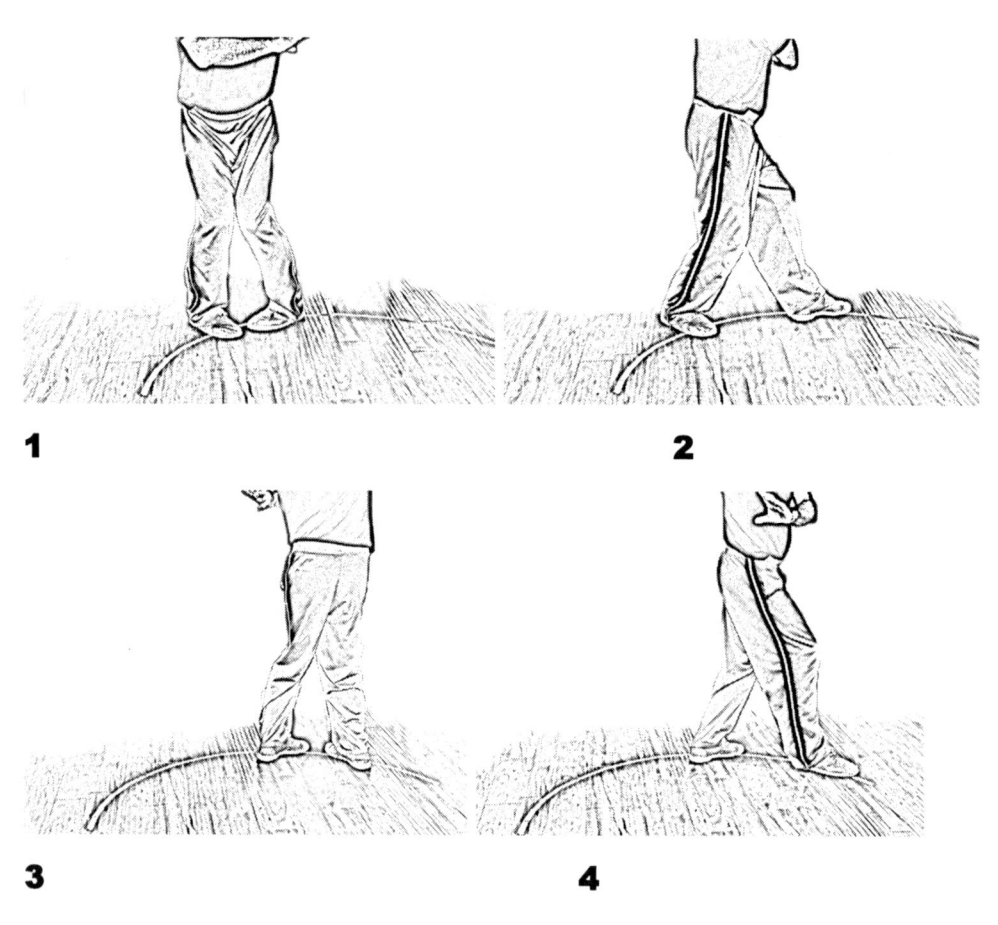

3　　　　　　　　　　　　　　**4**

Four-Step Turn

Training Tips

One of the difficulties students have initially is conceptualizing that we cannot really walk **exactly on** the circle. The nature of taking eight steps with our feet is that although the feet have a natural curve, they are somewhat rectangular in shape and thus do not exactly match the curve of a circle. Therefore walking an eight step circle consists of putting eight essentially straight segments (the feet) onto a circle

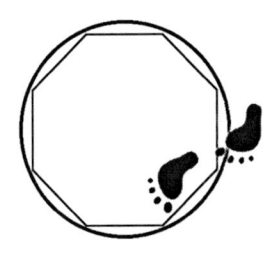

When walking the circle using Kou Bu and Bai Bu **the heels are never on a line.** This means that if you are walking clockwise and your left foot has just hooked (Kou Bu), and you pivot on the left heel to make the foot go straight the left heel should be on one side of an imaginary line running between the two feet and the right heel should be on the other side of the imaginary line. This is diagramed below.

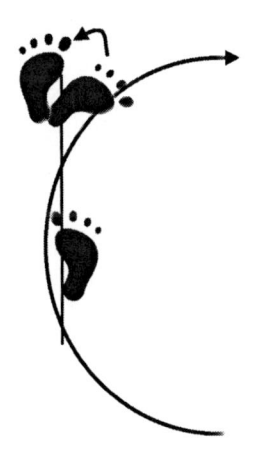

If the heels are on a line, the body is unstable and off balance. This is good way to check your posture as you progress to more complex steps. Simply turn the toes of the feet to face the same direction and see if there is a bit of space between your heels.

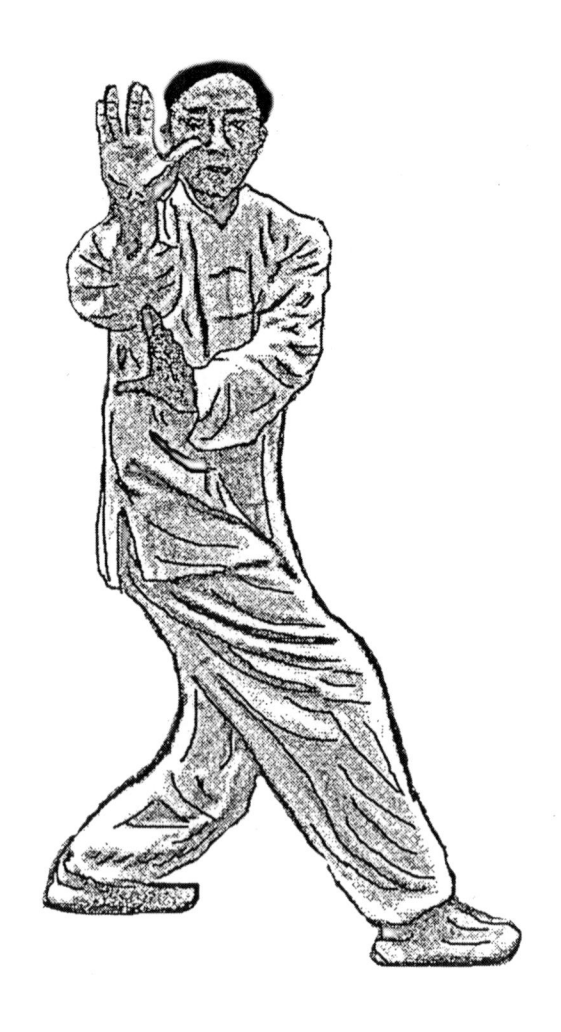

Millstone Pushing Posture
A drawing from a photo of Zhao Da Yuan from the Pa Kua Chang Journal Vol.3, No. 3 March/April 1993. Pacific Grove, CA: High View Publications.

Chapter 6
The Eight Palms of Ding Shi

Once you have practiced walking the circle and changing direction with the Downward Sinking Palm, the other seven body patterns can be added one by one. The stepping and turning pattern will be the same, but the body configuration will be different. In all eight postures it is important to maintain the body alignments outlined in the previous chapter, while incorporating the new alignments specific to each posture. Make sure that you are not twisting the spine in order to turn toward the center of the circle. Instead fold the kua to help you open the Mingmen point and turn the yao. This will aid the opening action of the channels and collaterals and prevent any binding of the vertebrae.

Kidney Breathing

Regulation of the breath is an essential element in the practice of Nei Gong. Because the vital force and the breath are interlinked, breathing correctly, naturally and easily immeasurably aids the functioning of the internal organs and the movement of the vital force through the jing luo. Deep diaphragmatic or "Kidney Breathing" is the breathing you will be performing while walking the circle holding the eight Ding Shi postures.

With the body alignments set and the mind focused on the breath, bring your attention to the *Dan Tian*. For our purposes, **the *Dan Tian* is the general area between the navel and the pubic bone. It is not on the surface of the body, but located just in front of the spine.**

- Breathe naturally and deeply, feeling the lower abdomen expand with each inhalation.

- Feel the area in your back that is directly behind the Dan Tian also expanding.
- The **whole** Dan Tian area, front, back and sides expands and contracts with each breath.
- Let the breath sink down and back into the sacrum and the kidneys.
- Do not force the air in, but let it naturally and smoothly flow inward.
- Remember that inhaling is effortless: the diaphragm drops creating a negative air pressure inside the lungs. This **allows** the air outside to enter and sink inward and downward.
- When you exhale, mentally observe or feel the breath rise and move up and out through the nose.
- The breath is like a winding thread or a gentle stream that moves evenly and smoothly down to fill the Dan Tian and up to be exhaled.
- Again pay attention to the smooth flow of air and its passage in and out of the body. See if you can observe the entire movement of the breath from the moment it enters the body to the finish of the exhale.

Kidney Breathing cannot be forced by pushing the air in and forcing the lower abdomen to expand. **Simply focus your attention on the Dan Tian and the Qi/Breath will follow**. Over time, simply by focusing you attention in this way the breathing will naturally slow, become deeper, longer, smoother and even. Like sediment sinking to the bottom of a pool of water, Qi/Breath will sink to the lower abdomen. Just as the sediment sinks naturally and without effort to the bottom of the pool, the Qi/Breath will also sink without physical effort. With practice, your breathing will automatically become:

Natural - Easy and unforced
Slow - Unhurried

Deep - Like a bellows, filling completely and fully

Long - Like drawing a thread through cloth

Smooth - Uninterrupted and continuous

Even - Inhalation and exhalation are even and equal in force

The Magpie Bridges

Although this was mentioned in the previous chapter, it is important to reiterate the importance of lifting the perineum and touching the tip of the tongue to the upper palate. This connects the upper and lower "magpie gates" which act almost like circuit breakers for the flow of vital force through the central channel – Ren Mai, Du Mai and Chong Mai. Without the circuit being activated, it is difficult for these channels to open up properly.

The Lao Gong Point

Energetically the acu-point at the center of the palm – *Lao Gong* "Palace of Labor" (Pericardium 8) - has a connection with the Yong Quan point on the foot. As you walk let some of your attention go to the center of the palm. Keep the palm centers hollow and "empty". With each step you may feel an energetic pulse that moves from palm to palm. If you do not notice this, don't worry. As the stepping and circling become more natural, it will happen automatically.

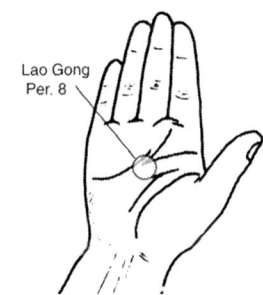

Lao Gong
Per. 8

Changing Direction on the Circle: An Alternative Method

In the previous chapter you learned a four-step turn to change direction. An alternative method is to turn with two steps. When walking clockwise, Kou Bu (hook step) with left (outside) foot. As the weight shifts to the left foot, let the right foot swing in a Bai Bu step, turning you rightward to face in the opposite direction. As the right foot completes its step, it makes a slight Kou Bu which begins to turn the body left, rotating you toward the center of the circle as you begin to walk counter-clockwise.

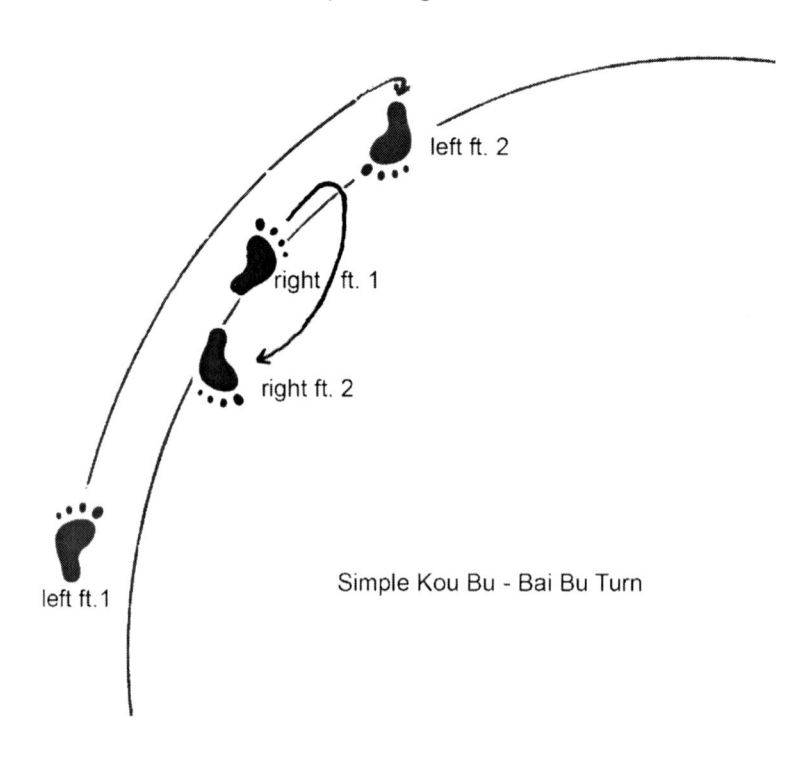

left ft. 2

right ft. 1

right ft. 2

left ft. 1

Simple Kou Bu - Bai Bu Turn

The Eight Ding Shi Palms

Although later the eight Ding Shi palms can be performed in various orders and combinations, in the beginning you should practice them in the order they are presented below. Walk for 1-3 minutes in one direction with each palm and then change directions and walk for another 1-3 minutes with the same palm. Then change directions and proceed to the next palm. In this way a practice session can take anywhere from 15-16 minutes to one hour.

Important!

Practice time should be relative to your constitution, requirements and ability to perform the *Ding Shi* correctly. There is no point in forcing yourself to walk for an hour if you are tense and uncomfortable for most of the practice session. The body should be relaxed and without strain; the footwork stable and smooth. This will not happen all at once, so time should be increased gradually. On days when you are very fatigued or not feeling well do less. Women should practice for shorter time periods when they are menstruating.

How to Begin Practice

Always start with the Downward Sinking Palm. Begin with the feet together. Inhale and raise the arms to the sides. As they reach the level of the crown, fold the arms inward and exhale as you press downward with the palms until they reach the level of the hips. Simultaneously, as the arms descend, the inside foot steps out onto the circle and the body turns in toward the inside of the circle by folding and sitting the kua. As the hands press down let the breath and intention sink with them.

Downward Sinking Palm

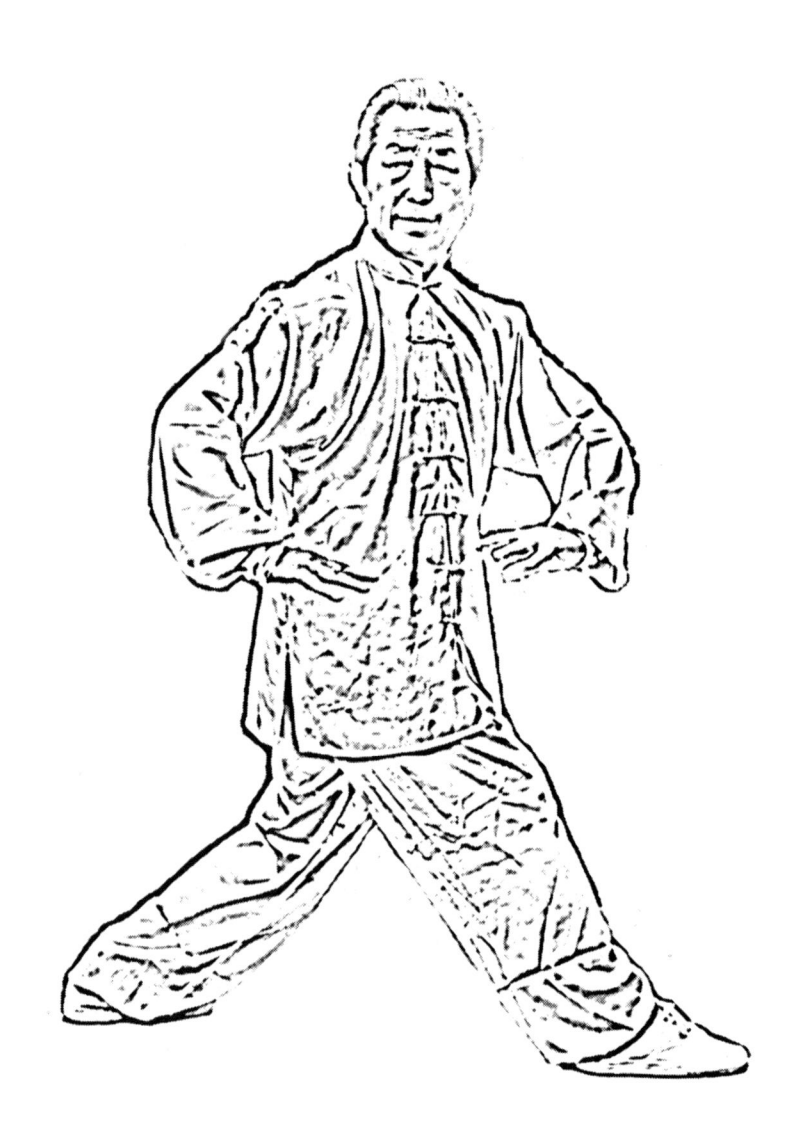

Downward Sinking Palm
Drawing from a photo of Gao Ji Wu taken by Valerie Ghent

Downward Sinking Palm

- Sink the palms downward and as you rotate the arms inward, let the chest and shoulders round slightly. There is a feeling of space in each armpit.
- The fingertips of both hands point inward to face each other while the thumbs point at the two kua.
- Internally the palms rotate inward and move toward each other while simultaneously there is a feeling of them rotating outward and pulling apart. These two forces balance each other so that the body feels relaxed and supple, yet loaded like a coiled spring.
- It should feel as though you are pushing a ball down gently into the water.
- The sinking of the arms is a function of the sinking of the tailbone and sacrum opposed by the uplifting of the head and upper back. This is aided by sitting the kua and bending the knees so the weight falls through the yongquan acu-point – simultaneously there is an internal feeling of straightening through the knees and pushing upward from the soles of the feet. These forces also balance and cancel each other.
- Slacken and sink the shoulders to help the elbows extend naturally.
- Empty the chest, lift up the upper back and sink the lower back.
- Twist the kua inward and close the knees as you walk the circle.
- The fingers of each hand are separate and the palm center is hollow. The hands assume the shape of the "tile palm" (see general body alignment #4 in Chapter 4).

Training Tip

In some styles of Ba Gua Zhang, the Downward Sinking Palm is referred to as "The Tiger Descends the Mountain." If your alignments are correct when walking the circle using this palm configuration, it can feel internally as though your hands are grasping the ground like a tiger walking down a hill.

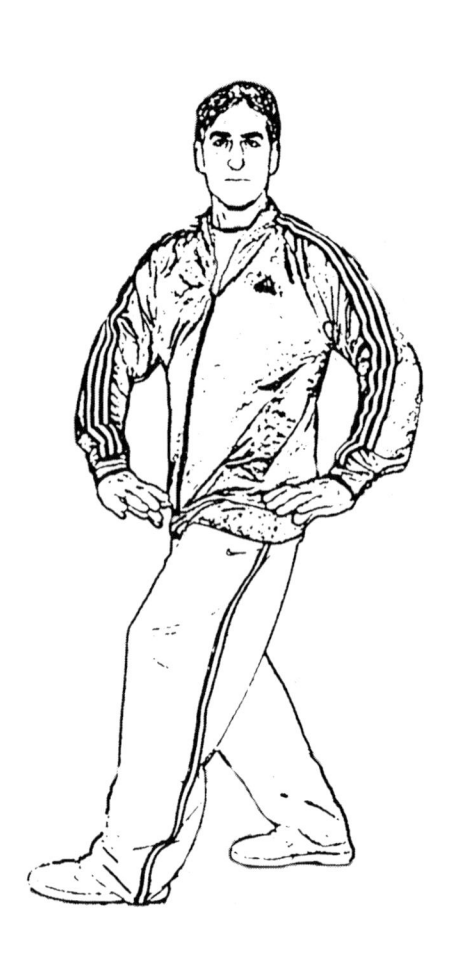

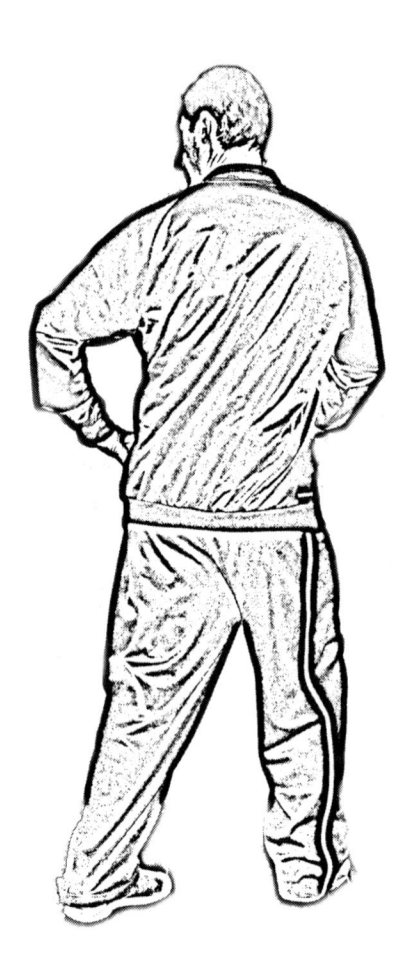

Heaven Upholding Palm

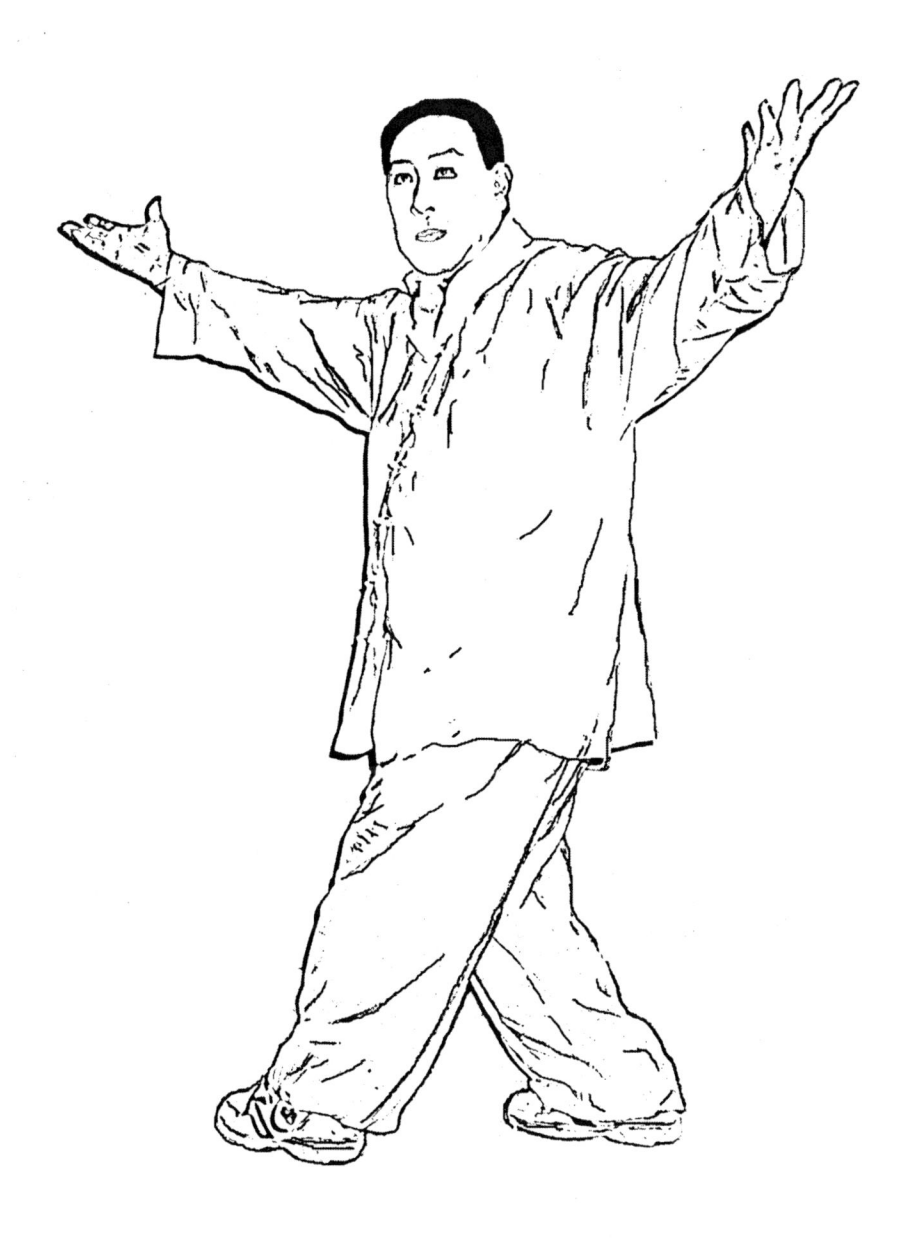

Heaven Upholding Palm
Drawing from an author photo of Zhang Hua Sen

Heaven Upholding Palm

- From the Downward Sinking Palm position, bring the hands upward towards the chest, leading with the fingertips. Then push outward and upwards as the palm simultaneously pierce outward and lift upwards.
- The arms extend outward and upward as though simultaneously upholding plates or objects and penetrating through something.
- The fingers of each hand are separate and the palm center is hollow. The hands assume the shape of the "tile palm."
- The elbows sink and the shoulder loosens and relaxes. The arms are in the shape of a bow.
- The hands raise slightly higher than the shoulders. The raising action of the arms comes from the back and ribs rather than the shoulder muscles. It is assisted by raising the vertex and the upper back, sinking the tail and sitting the kua, all of which balance the uplifting motion.
- The arms and chest form a gentle concave curve. The two arms therefore form less than a 180 degree angle. The alignment of the chest and the arms sets the hand just in front of the shoulders.
- If the arms raise too high you will feel unstable. If they do not lift enough it will feel as though you are collapsing.
- The arm that faces the inside of the circle will not point exactly toward the center of the circle, but will point slightly behind the center of the circle and the direction you are walking in.

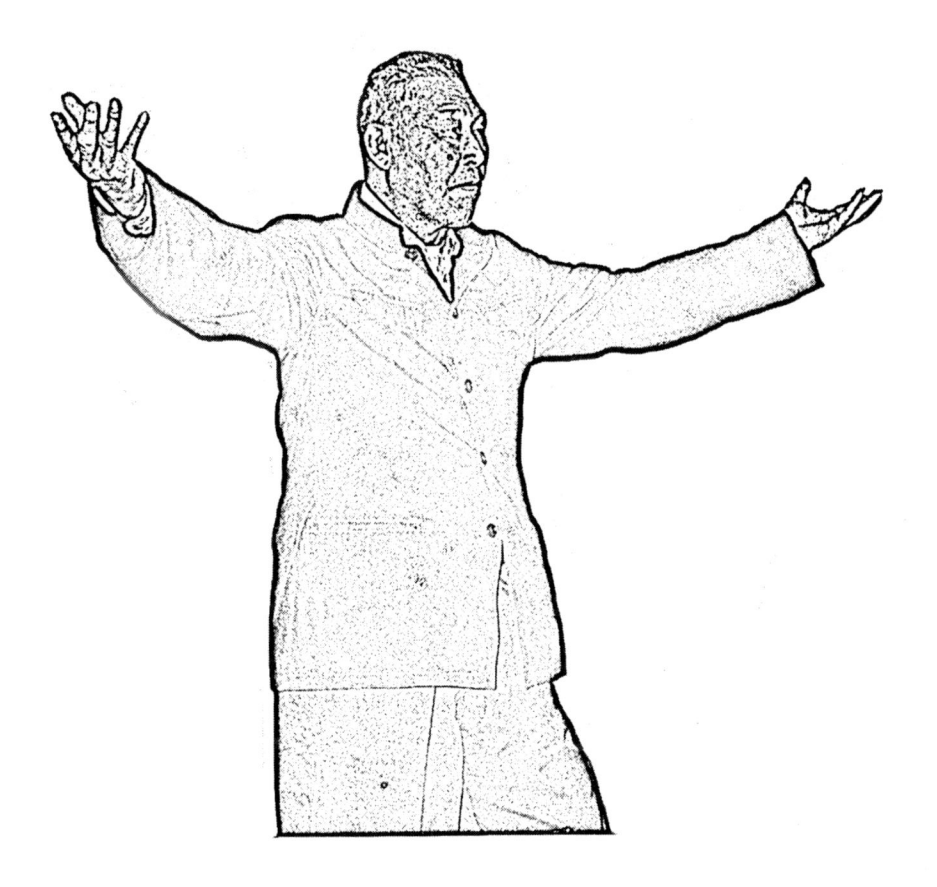

Heaven Upholding Palm
Drawing from an author photo of Wang Shi Tong

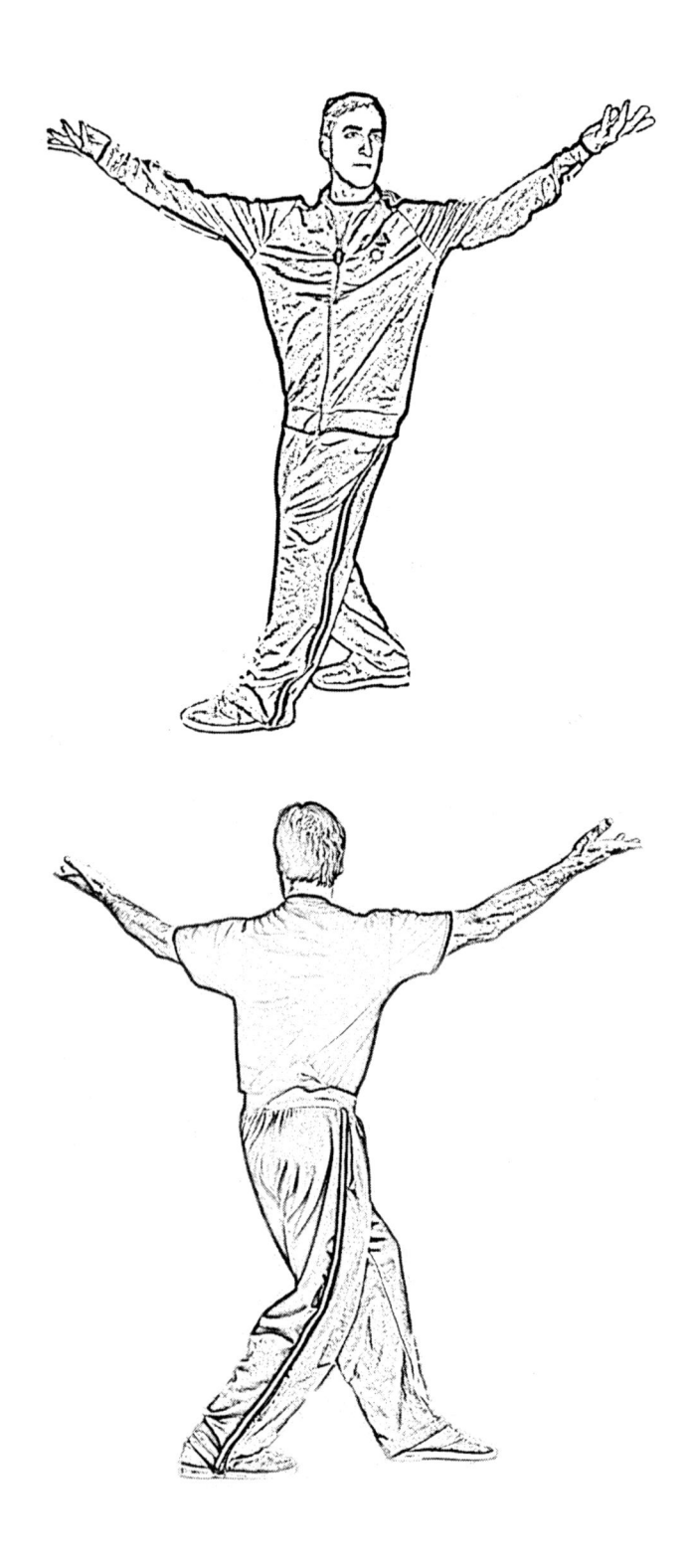

Moon Embracing Palm

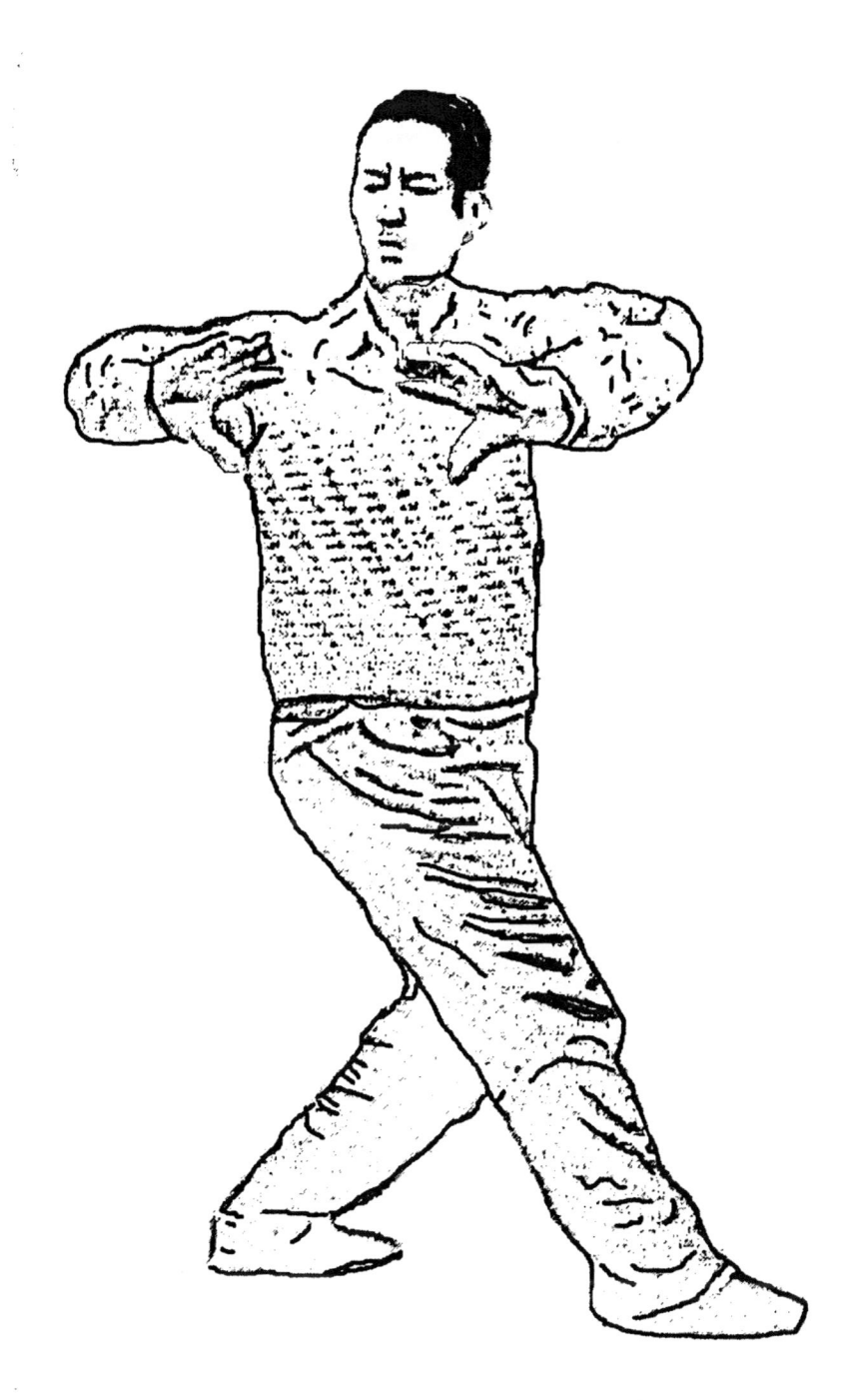

Moon Embracing Palm
Drawing from a photo of Cheng De Liang from the Ba Gua Chang Journal
Vol.6, No. 1 Nov/Dec 1995. Pacific Grove, CA: High View Publications.

Moon Embracing Palm

- From the previous posture push the palms outward as the thumbs drop downward.
- The hands are at the height of the shoulder and there is a quality of embracing something.
- The hands push outward as if protecting the chest.
- The chest is relaxed and the back tightens slightly as the elbows extend to push the palms forward.
- Loosen and relax the shoulders and feel as though the shoulder blades are glued down or "buttoned" to the ribs.
- The fingers are slightly separated and the palm centers are hollow.
- The fingertips, hands and arms feel as though they are drawn towards each other, yet at the same time they feel as though they are moving apart; as though they are pulling something apart.
- As you walk and rotate, it should feel as though you are simultaneously embracing something and pushing something ahead of you.
- Other names for this palm are the Mountain Pushing Palm and the Double Bumping Palm. Both convey the image of pushing or bumping something with the palms.

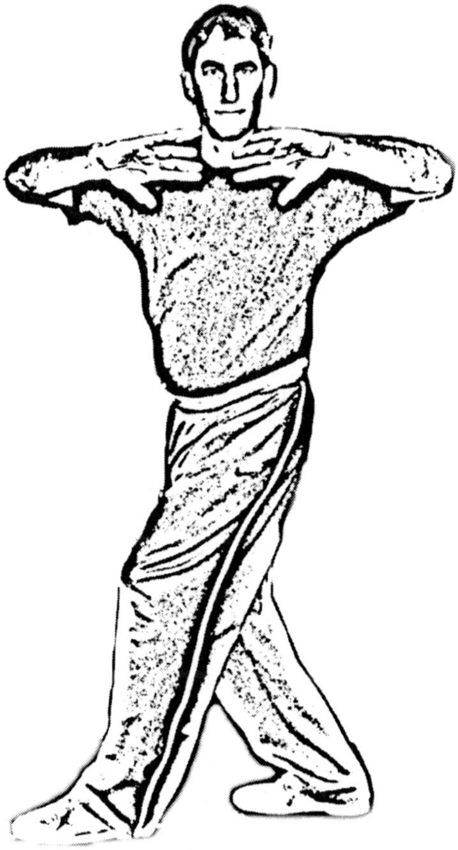

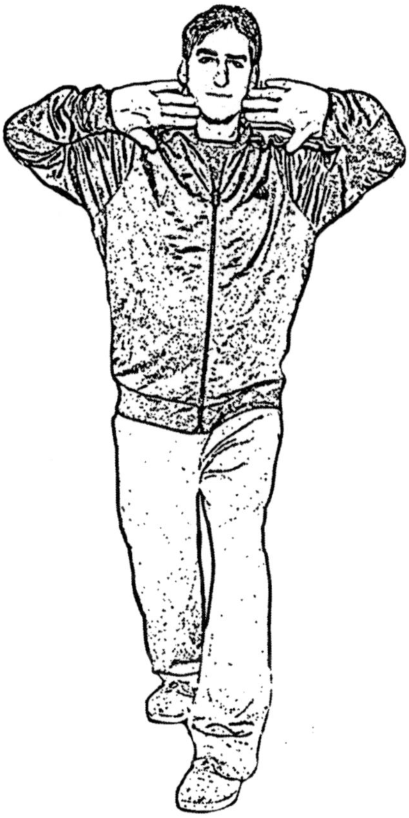

Ball Rolling Palm

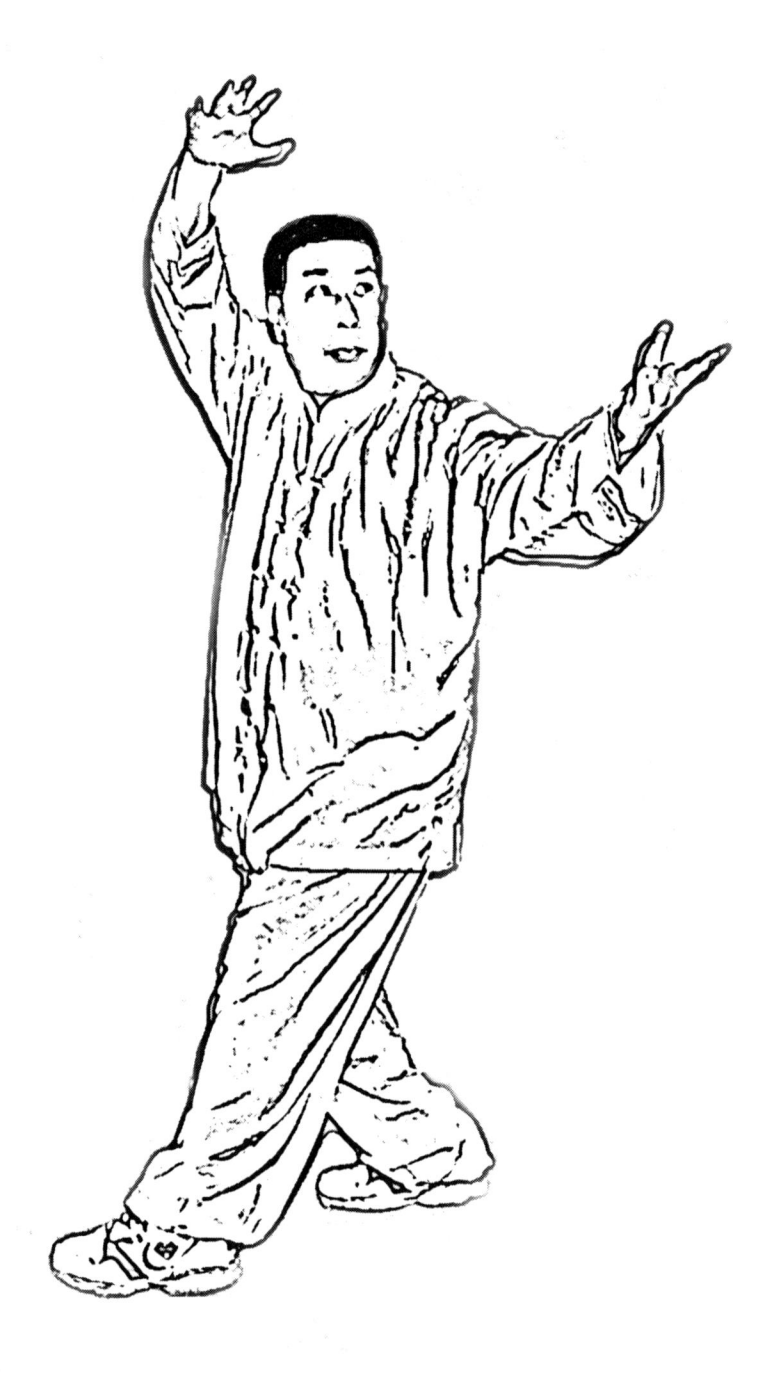

Ball Rolling Palm
Drawing from an author photo of Zhang Hua Sen

Ball Rolling Palm

- The two hands and arms feel like they are holding a ball.
- The two palms combine as you turn with a feeling of embracing or holding the yao (back and waist).
- The back is round and the upper (outside) arm creates a faint tugging sensation in the lower back, which in turn feels like it pulls the leg forward.
- The shoulders are dropped and loosened and ribs extend forward.
- Keep the shoulders level and cultivate a regal quality by erecting the head with a feeling of prestige.
- The palm centers are hollow and empty as though conforming to the shape of a ball.
- The side of the body stretches forward to walk the circle and the high (outside) hand helps pull the steps.
- Create a feeling of roundness in the body. Feel like your hands are holding a ball as you walk and turn, but also that part of the ball is composed of the chest and back themselves.
- This posture is sometimes called Lion Holds the Ball.

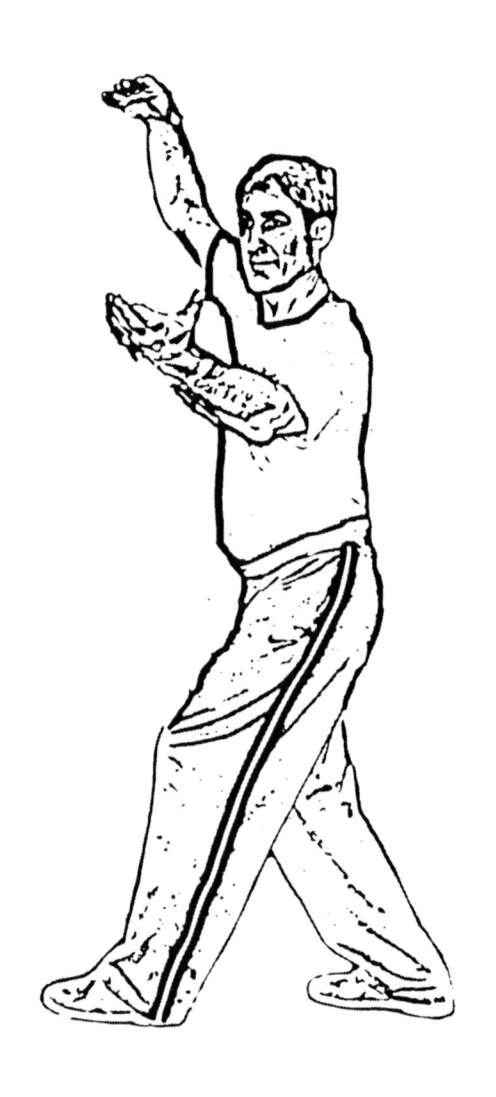

Spear Upholding Palm

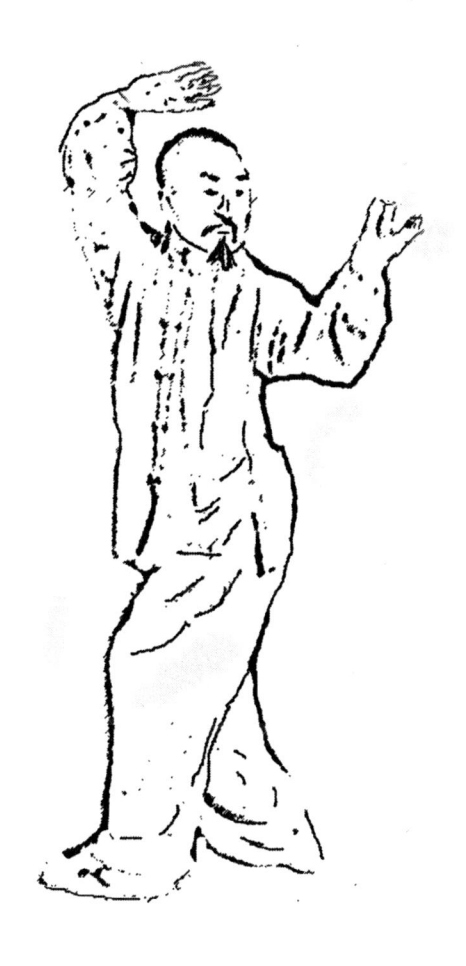

Spear Upholding Palm
A drawing from a photo of Sha Guo Zheng from the Ba Gua Chang Journal, Vol.6, No. 1 Nov/Dec 1995. Pacific Grove, CA: High View Publications.

Spear Upholding Palm

- The inside hand extends outward palm up, while the palm of the outside hand extends forward and outward in a curved shape at the height of the head.
- The outside hand pulls the side forward and pulls the step.
- Extend the strength outward through the ribs and arms as the yao and central channel turn the body.
- Sitting the *kua* aids the hands in pushing forward and extending.
- The shoulders relax and loosen and both shoulders and elbows sink.
- The palms take the shape of the tile palm.
- This palm takes its name from a Ba Gua method of using the spear.

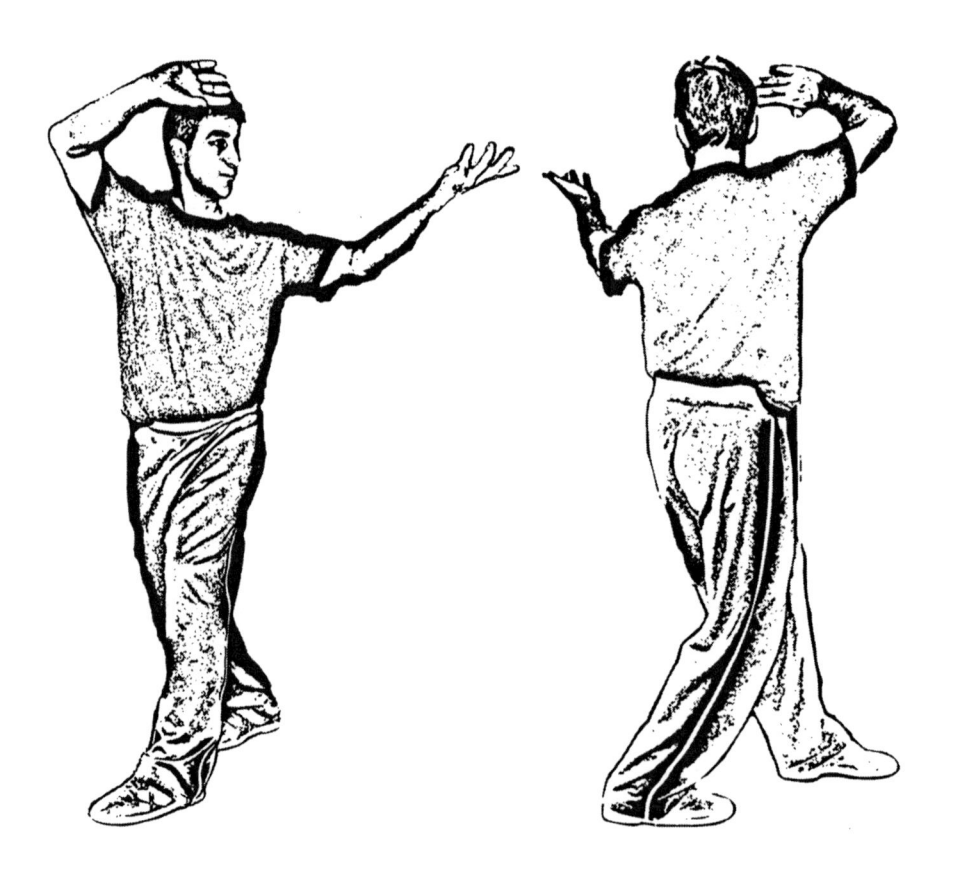

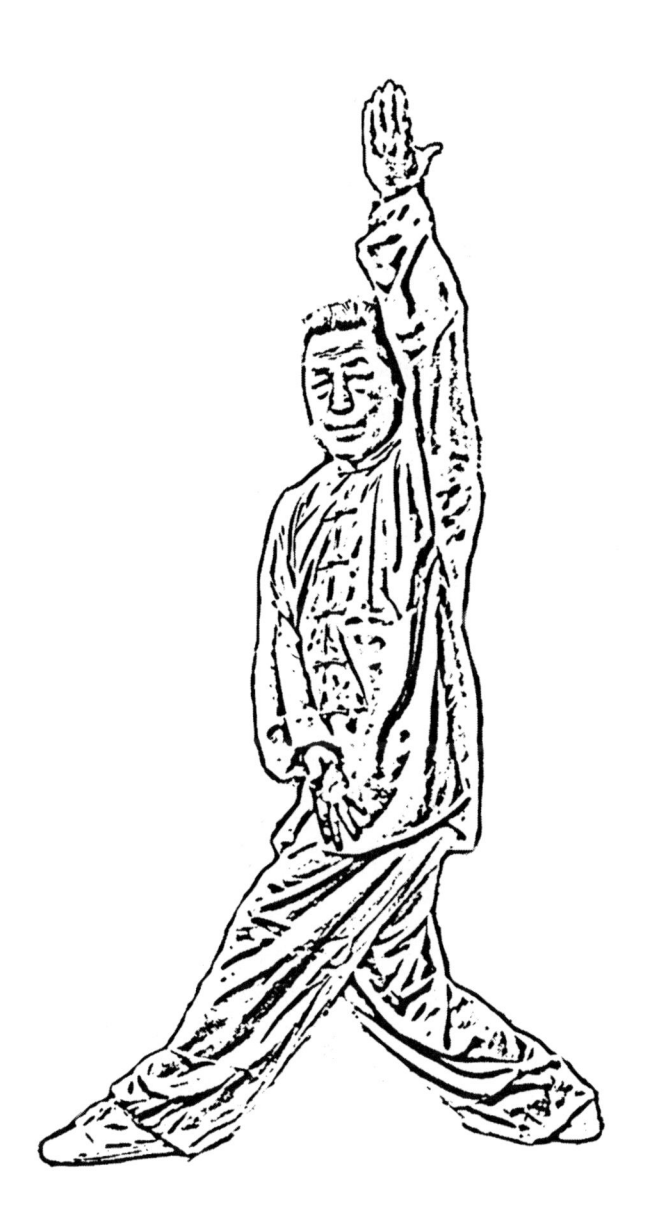

Heaven Pointing Ground Drawing Palm

Heaven Pointing Ground Drawing Palm
Drawing from a photo of Gao Ji Wu taken by Valerie Ghent

Heaven Pointing Ground Drawing Palm

- The inside hand drills and extends upward with the palm facing backward to "point at heaven," while the outside hand pierces downward toward the center of the circle facing forward to "draw on the ground."
- The opposing forces of the two palms and the two sides of the body create a twist that goes from the sole of the foot through the whole body.
- The shoulders relax and drop.
- Slacken the yao (low back and waist) to stretch the arms.
- Sit down and fold the kua to help the arms pierce and drill.
- Slackening the yao and sitting the kua makes the steps smooth as though they are sweeping the ground
- The hands follow the spiral of the arms to form the tile palm.
- The eyes look past the upper arm (inside arm) toward the inside of the circle.

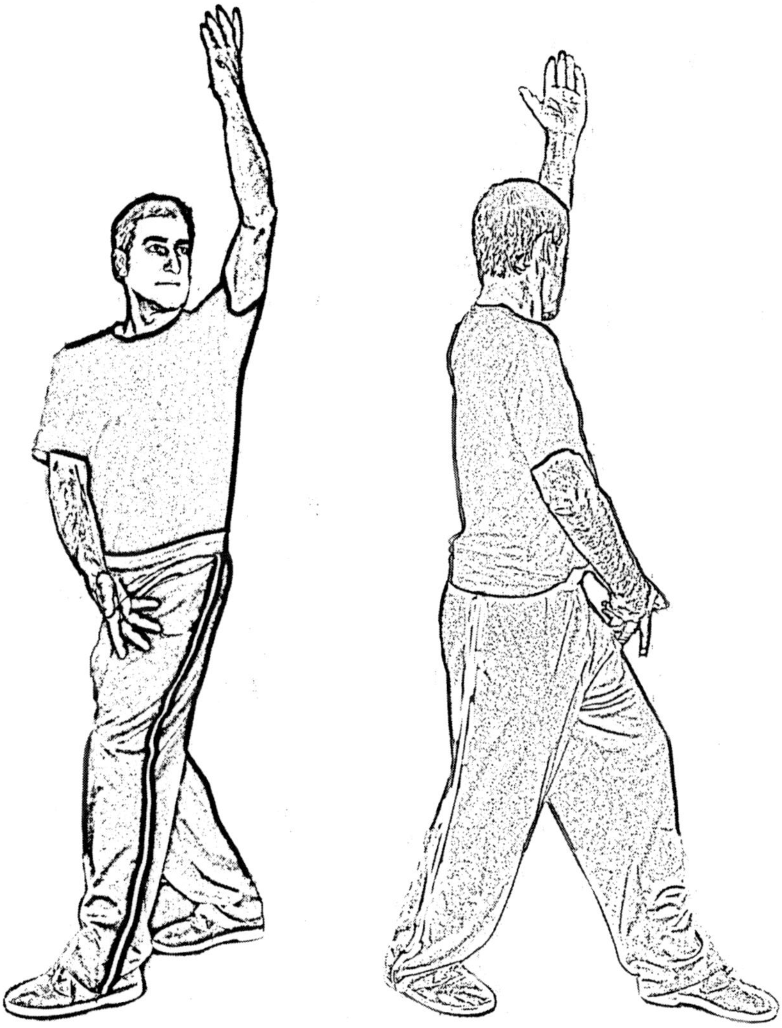

Yin Yang Fish Palm

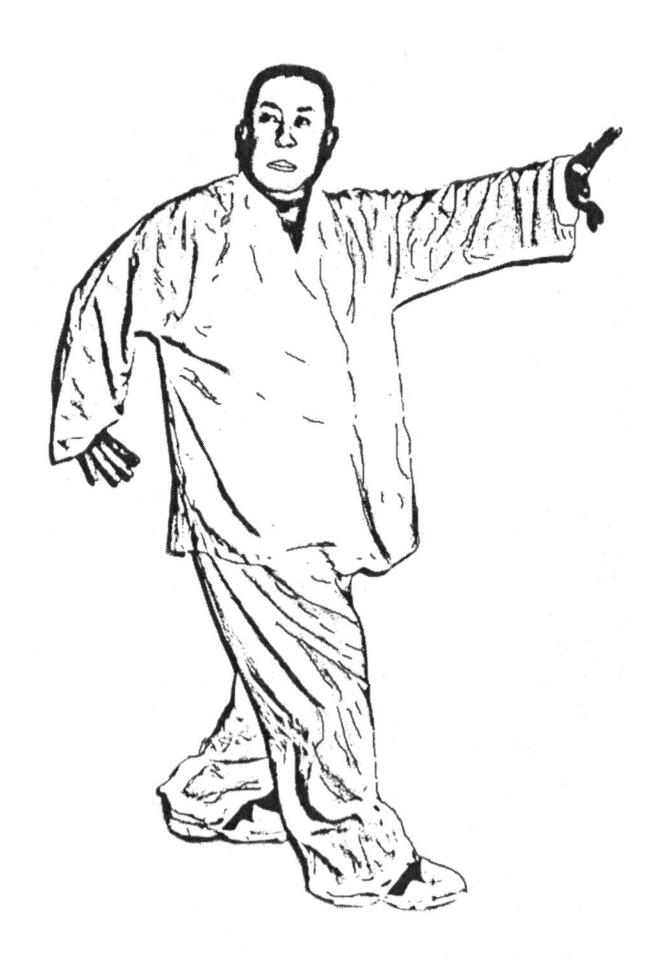

Yin Yang Fish Palm
Drawing from an author photo of Zhang Hua Sen

Yin Yang Fish Palm

- The arms and body make a yin-yang shape.
- The outside hand curves toward the inside of the circle, while the inside hand wraps behind the back opposite Ming Men (the middle of the lower back).
- The outside hand follows the curve of the circle while the inside hand pushes away from the body.
- Extend the strength outward through the ribs and arms as the yao, waist and central channel turn the body.
- The back is taut and the chest is empty and relaxed.
- Let the curved body shape aid the steps.
- Fingers are apart and the palms are hollow.

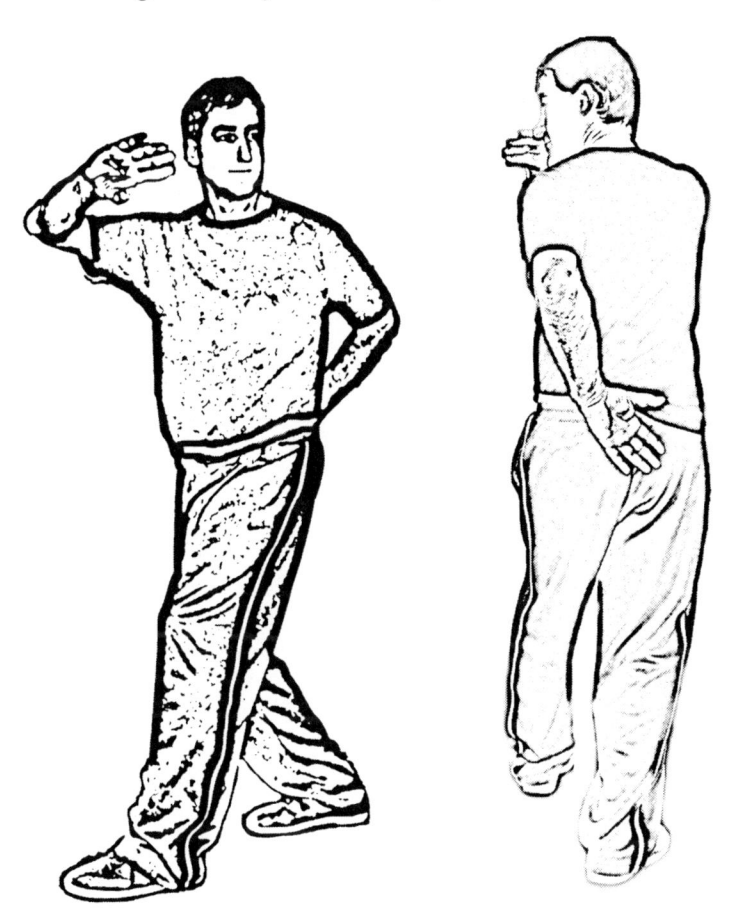

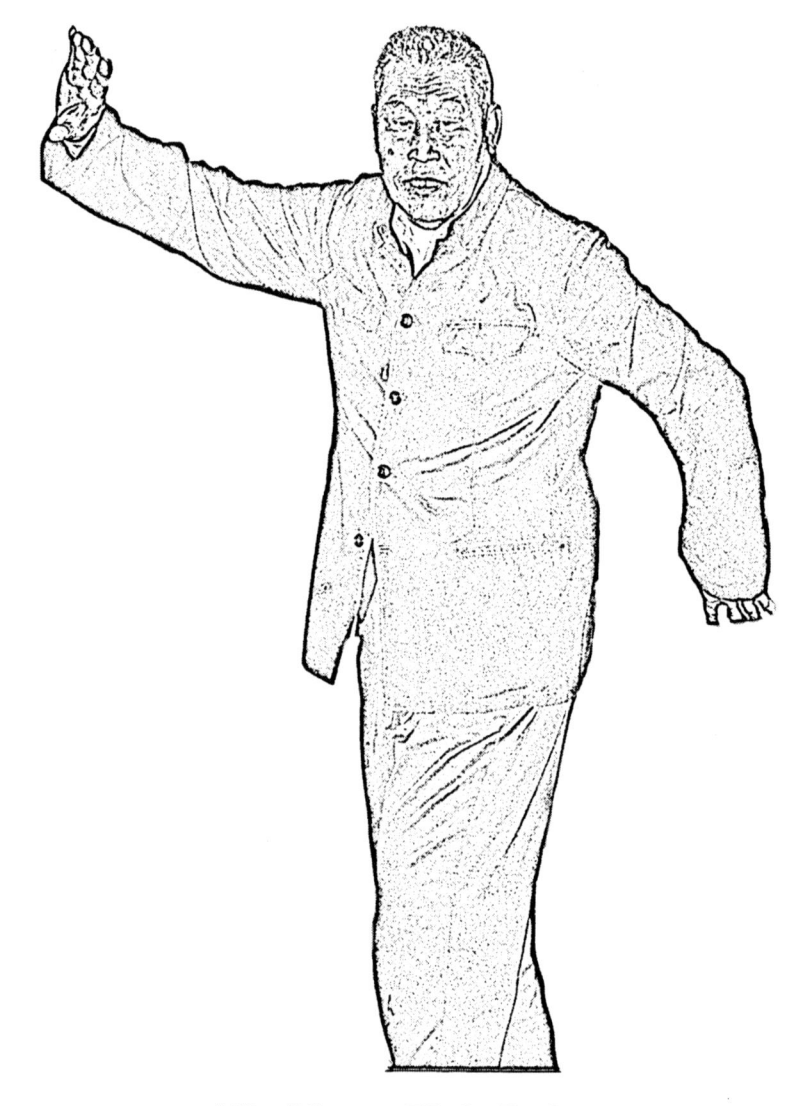

Yin Yang Fish Palm
Drawing from an author photo of Wang Shi Tong

Millstone Pushing Palm

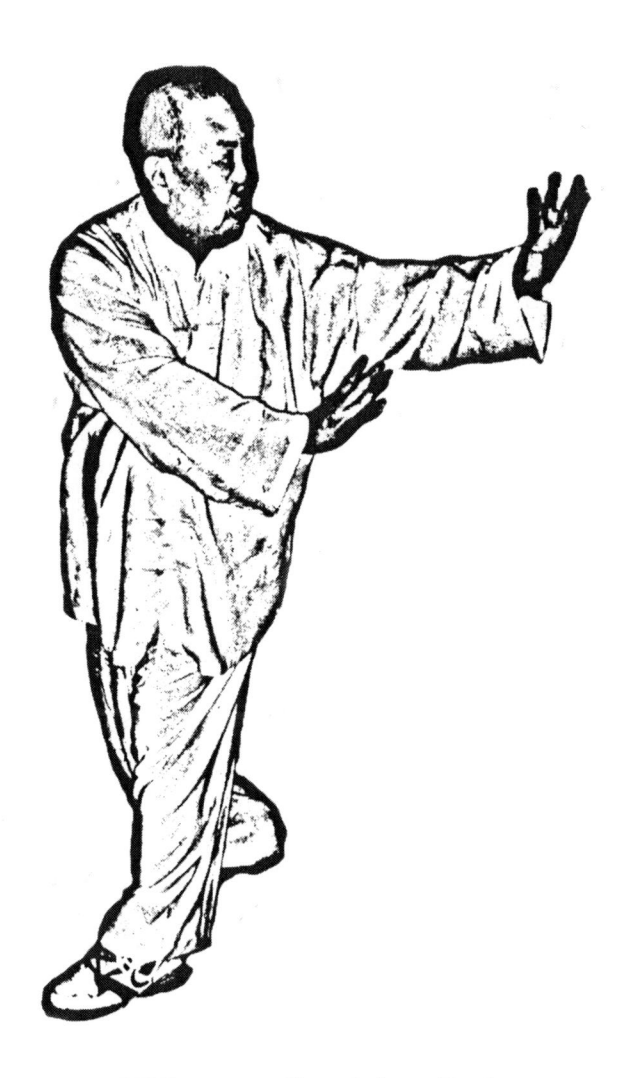

Millstone Pushing Palm
Drawing from an author photo of Zhang Hua Sen

Millstone Pushing Palm

- The fingers of the inside hand point upward at the level of the eyebrow and the palm root drops downward.
- The outside arm has a wrapping, embracing force. It wraps around the body so that the fingers point at the elbow of the inside arm.
- The palms take the shape of the tile palm.
- There is space under the armpits and the elbows drop down as though protecting the body.
- There is a feeling of extending through the arms, yet the wrists and elbows remain supple.
- The reaching and extending of the outside arm helps drive the steps.
- The arms are curved. They are not sharply bent or straight.
- The shoulder blades are buttoned down and "glued" to the ribs.
- The arms have a twisting wrapping force.
- The outside hand is reaching toward the elbow of the inside hand.
- The kua sits and twists and the body turns so that when the inside foot is forward, the inside hand is in line with the rear (outside foot).

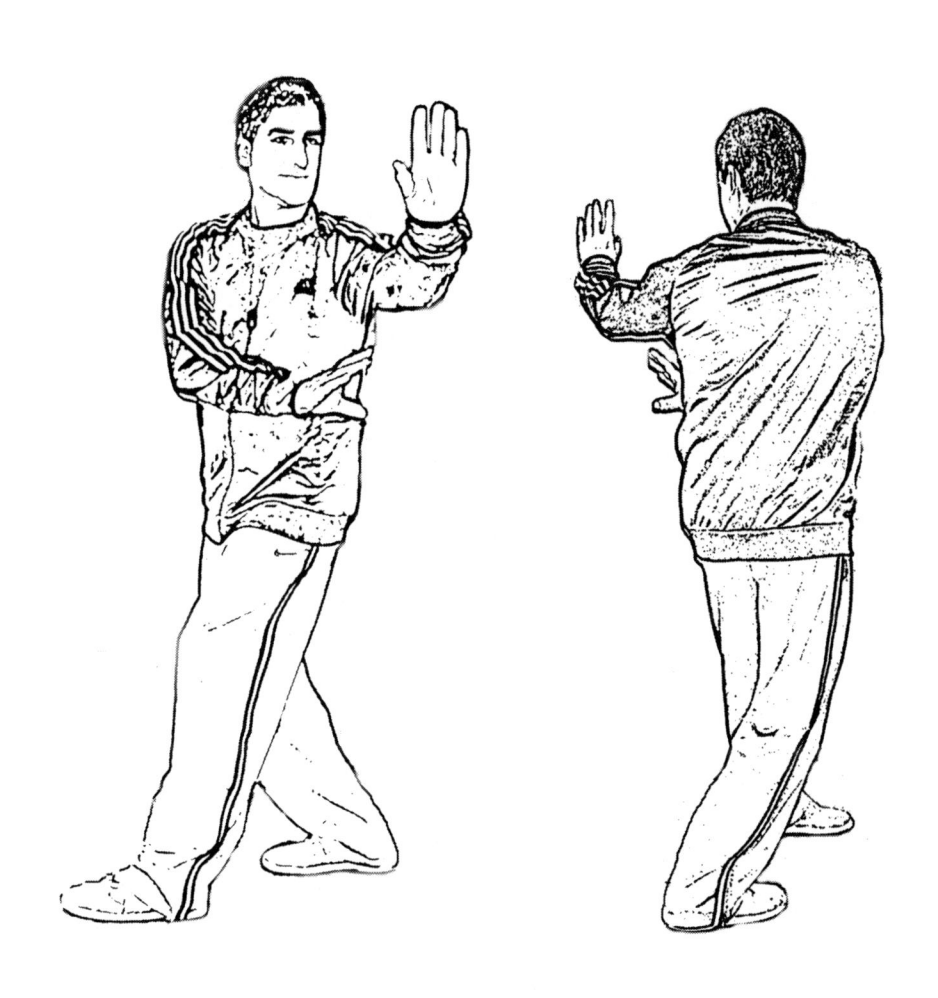

Peach Offering Palm

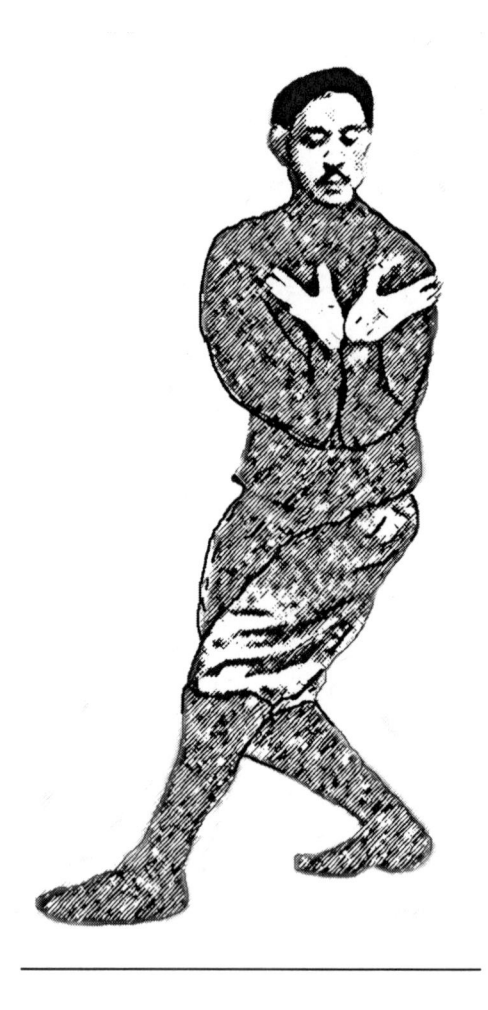

Peach Offering Palm or Double Embracing Palm

Drawing from a photo of Sun Xi Kun from the Ba Gua Chang Journal Vol.6, No. 1 Nov/Dec 1995. Pacific Grove, CA: High View Publications.

Peach Offering Palm/Double Embracing Palm

- The elbows are brought inward and upward so that the back expands.
- The inward and upward action is like offering something.
- The arms twist and wrap inward and the palms spiral upward.
- The palms touch and the fingers open like a flower unfolding its petals
- The chest is relaxed and empty and the shoulders drop downward.
- The back opens and curves and Ming Men spreads and opens.
- The kua sits and the body crouches.

Note: This ninth palm is not standard in this method of Ba Gua Zhang, but is included here because it is sometimes added as a transitional movement between some of the other palms, and because it has its own unique properties (see Chapter 9).

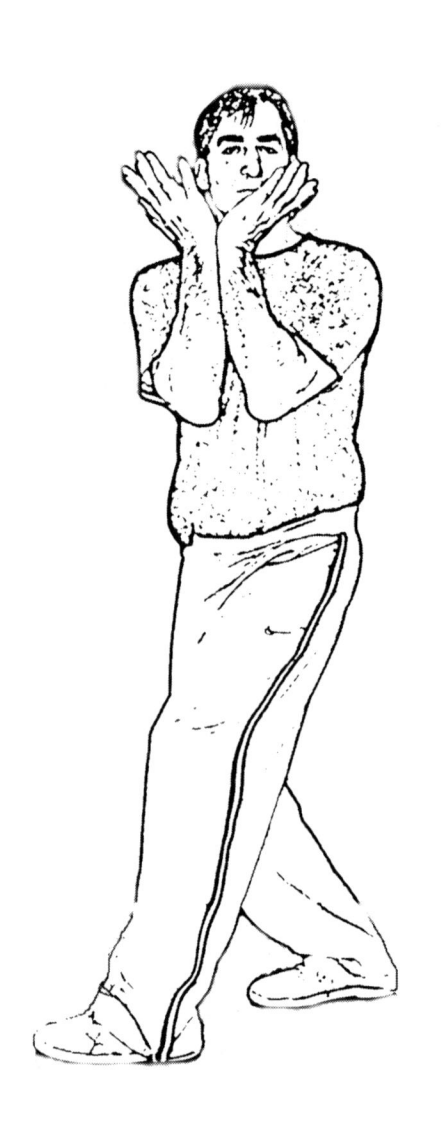

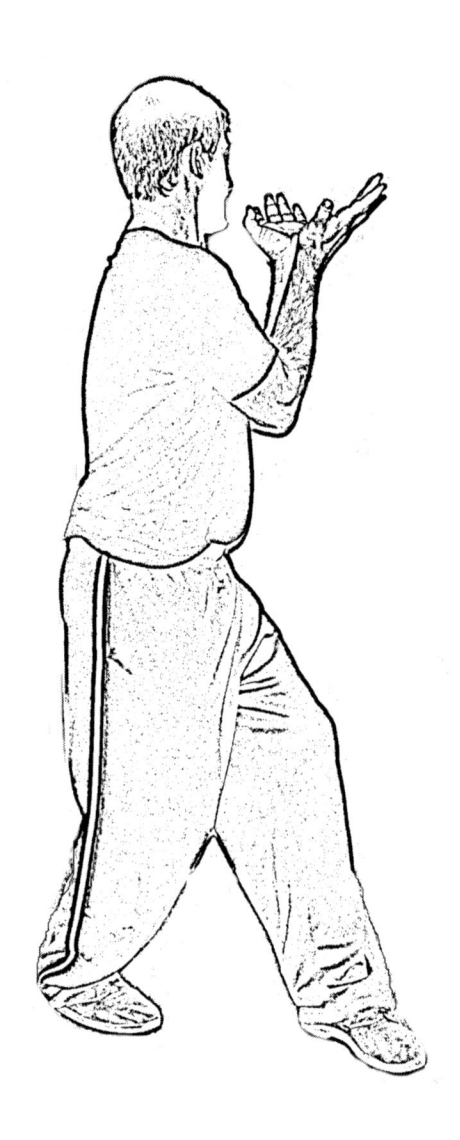

Chapter 7
The Six Yin and Yang Axes

The Six Axes: Twelve Primary Channels

There are 365 acupuncture points located on the "fourteen meridians". The fourteen meridians in this context consist of the twelve primary meridians and the Ren and Du channels – the only two of the eight extraordinary vessels that have their own distinct points. Although the twelve primary meridians (*Jing Zheng*) are distinctly labeled as separate, they can be more properly understood as six yin/yang energetic units, often known as the "six divisions" or "six levels". This division of these twelve channels into six energetic units tells us not only about their configuration and location, but also describes their interplay and movement.

At their most fundamental level, the channels and collaterals regulate yin and yang. The channels link, connect with and are expressions of the transformational processes that are themselves reflections of the unending transformation and interplay of yin and yang. Yang is expansive and outwardly moving, while yin is quiescent, a material expression of yang's motive force. Therefore an easy way to understand the meridians is to follow Joseph Helms in describing them as the Six Axes of the body.[44] These Six Energetic Axes are then further divided into three yang and three yin axes.

The Three Yang Axes are:

- Taiyang ("greater" or "highest" yang)
- Shaoyang ("lesser" or "younger" yang)
- Yangming (yang "brightness" or "radiance")

The Three Yin Axes are:

---

[44] *Acupuncture Energetics: A Clinical Approach for Physicians,* by Joseph M. Helms, Berkely CA: Medical Acupuncture Publishers, 1995.

- Taiyin ("greater" or "highest" yin)
- Shaoyin ("lesser" or "younger" yin)
- Jueyin ("terminal" or "absolute" yin)

The Meridians are named by three criteria:

1) Their association energetically with one of the six axis

2) Their connection through internal pathways to an internal organ or organs.

3) Their starting or ending point at the hand or foot

Taiyang:
- Bladder Channel (Foot Taiyang)
- Small Intestine Channel (Hand Taiyang)

Shaoyang
- Gallbladder Channel (Foot Shaoyang)
- Triple Heater Channel (Hand Shaoyang)

Yangming
- Stomach Channel (Foot Yangming)
- Large Intestine Channel (Hand Yangming)

Taiyin
- Spleen Channel (Foot Taiyin)
- Lung Channel (Hand Taiyin)

Shaoyin
- Kidney Channel (Foot Shaoyin)
- Heart Channel (Hand Shaoyin)

Jueyin
- Liver Channel (Foot Jueyin)
- Pericardium Channel (Hand Jueyin)

Inter-relationship and Movement of the Yin and Yang Axes

The 12 Regular Meridians of the arms and legs flow in the following pattern or circuit:

1. The yin meridians of the arms flow from the chest to the hand.
2. The yang meridians of the arms flow from the hands to the head.
3. The yang meridians of the legs flow from the head to the feet.
4. The yin meridians of the legs flow from the feet to the chest.

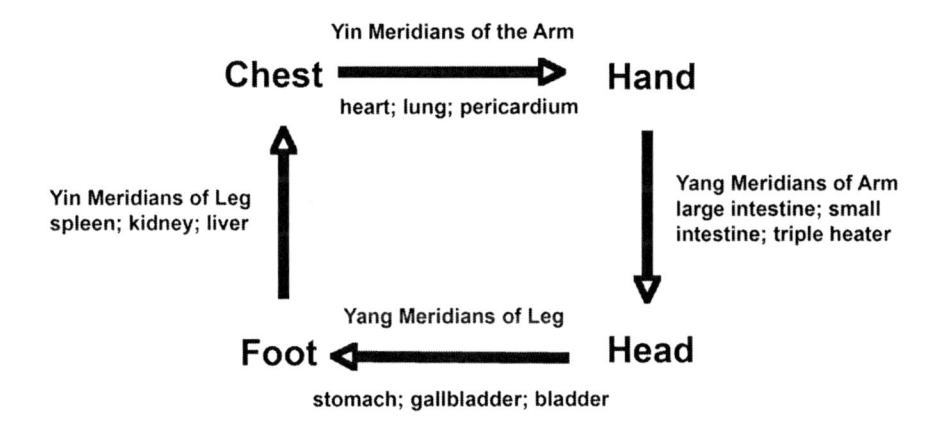

```
                    Yin Meridians of the Arm
         Chest ─────────────────▶ Hand
                  heart; lung; pericardium
           ▲                              │
           │                              │
  Yin Meridians of Leg          Yang Meridians of Arm
  spleen; kidney; liver         large intestine; small
                                intestine; triple heater
           │                              │
           │                              ▼
                    Yang Meridians of Leg
         Foot ◀───────────────── Head
                stomach; gallbladder; bladder
```

Inter-relationship & Movement of Yin and Yang Axes

In this way, the meridians then create four smaller circuits that are part of the larger circuit of all twelve. These circuits, their direction and order of circulation are diagrammed below:

Four Energetic Units/Circuits of the Six Axes

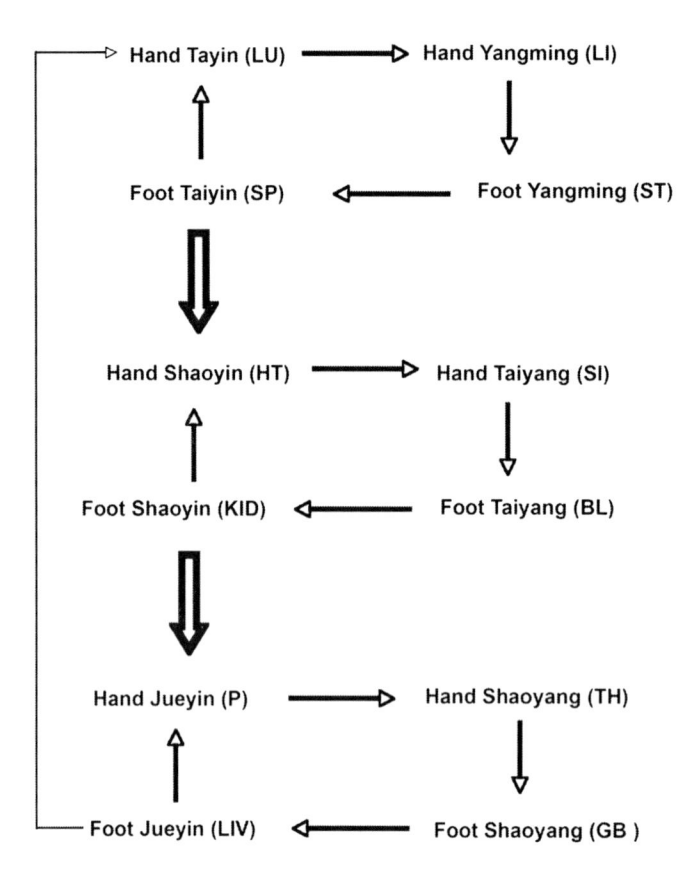

Hand Tayin (LU) → Hand Yangming (LI)

↑ ↓

Foot Taiyin (SP) ← Foot Yangming (ST)

⇓

Hand Shaoyin (HT) → Hand Taiyang (SI)

↑ ↓

Foot Shaoyin (KID) ← Foot Taiyang (BL)

⇓

Hand Jueyin (P) → Hand Shaoyang (TH)

↑ ↓

Foot Jueyin (LIV) ← Foot Shaoyang (GB)

This pattern of circulation is also evident in the circadian rhythm of the meridians. Below are the times each meridian is most active. It is least active in the opposite twelve hour period.

3 am - 5 am: Hand Taiyin - Lung (LU)

5 am - 7 am: Hand Yangming - Large Intestine (LI)

7 am - 9 am: Foot Yangming - Stomach (ST)

9 am - 11 am: Foot Taiyin - Spleen (SP)

11 am - 1 pm: Hand Shaoyin - Heart (HT)

1 pm - 3 pm: Hand Taiyang - Small Intestine (SI)

3 pm - 5 pm: Foot Taiyang - Bladder (BL)

5 pm - 7pm: Foot Shaoyin - Kidney (KID)

7 pm - 9 pm: Hand Jueyin - Pericardium (P)

9 pm - 11 pm: Hand Shaoyang   - San Jiao (SJ)

11pm - 1 am: Foot Taiyang   - Gallbladder (GB)

1 am – 3 am: Foot Jueyin - Liver (LIV)

The Three Movements: Open, Close and Pivot

Each of the six axes has a characteristic movement or way of operating within what is an ultimately unified system. These characteristic movements or actions tell us how each level or axis interacts with and regulates the fundamental yin and yang energies. The three movements are described are described as:

1. Open (*Kai*)
2. Close (*He*)
3. Pivot or Hinge (*Shu*)

Examining these three primal actions and their relationship to the six axes makes it easier to understand the meridians, their functioning and how they are modulated and activated through the practice of Ba Gua Circle Walking Nei Gong.

The Han dynasty text, *Huang Di Nei Jing* (The Yellow Emperor's Inner Cannon) is perhaps the fundamental doctrinal work in Chinese medicine. The *Nei Jing* describes the three yang and yin axes as follows:

Yang

Taiyang *controls the superficies (outer surface). It spreads yang qi to the exterior so it is open.*

Yang Ming *controls the interior. It receives yang qi to guard the viscera, so it is close.*

Shaoyang *is situated at the location located of half exterior and half interior to transport between the exterior and the interior, so it is pivot.*[45]

Yin

Taiyin *is at the superficies of the three yin; It is located in the middle to spread yin energy and irrigate its surroundings.*

Shaoyin *is the kidney. When the kidney energy is ample, the liver and spleen will bring their functions of open and close into full play; so it is the pivot.*

Jueyin *collects the yin energy and transmits it to the interior so it is close.*[46]

---

[45] *Yellow Emperor's Canon of Internal Medicine*, Bing Wang, translated by Nelson Liansheng Wu and Andrew Qi Wu. China Science and Technology Press, p. 46
[46] *Yellow Emperor's Canon of Internal Medicine*, Bing Wang, translated by Nelson Liansheng Wu and Andrew Qi Wu. China Science and Technology Press, p. 47.

Nguyen Van Nghi uses the analogy of a door to help conceptualize the functions of open, close and pivot.[47] The door may be closed to prevent the entry of unwelcome guests such as external pathogens, or to protect and support what is contained inside. But the door can also be opened to let in friends or positive nourishing influences. Whether the door opens (Taiyang and Taiyin) and closes (Yang Ming and Jueyin) well, depends largely on the hinges - the pivot point of the door (Shaoyang and Shaoyin). Only if the hinges function smoothly, can the energy circulate adequately.

---

[47] *Atlas of Acupuncture* by Claudia Focks. Churchill Livingstone (Elsevier Limited), 2008, p. 17.

Taiyang

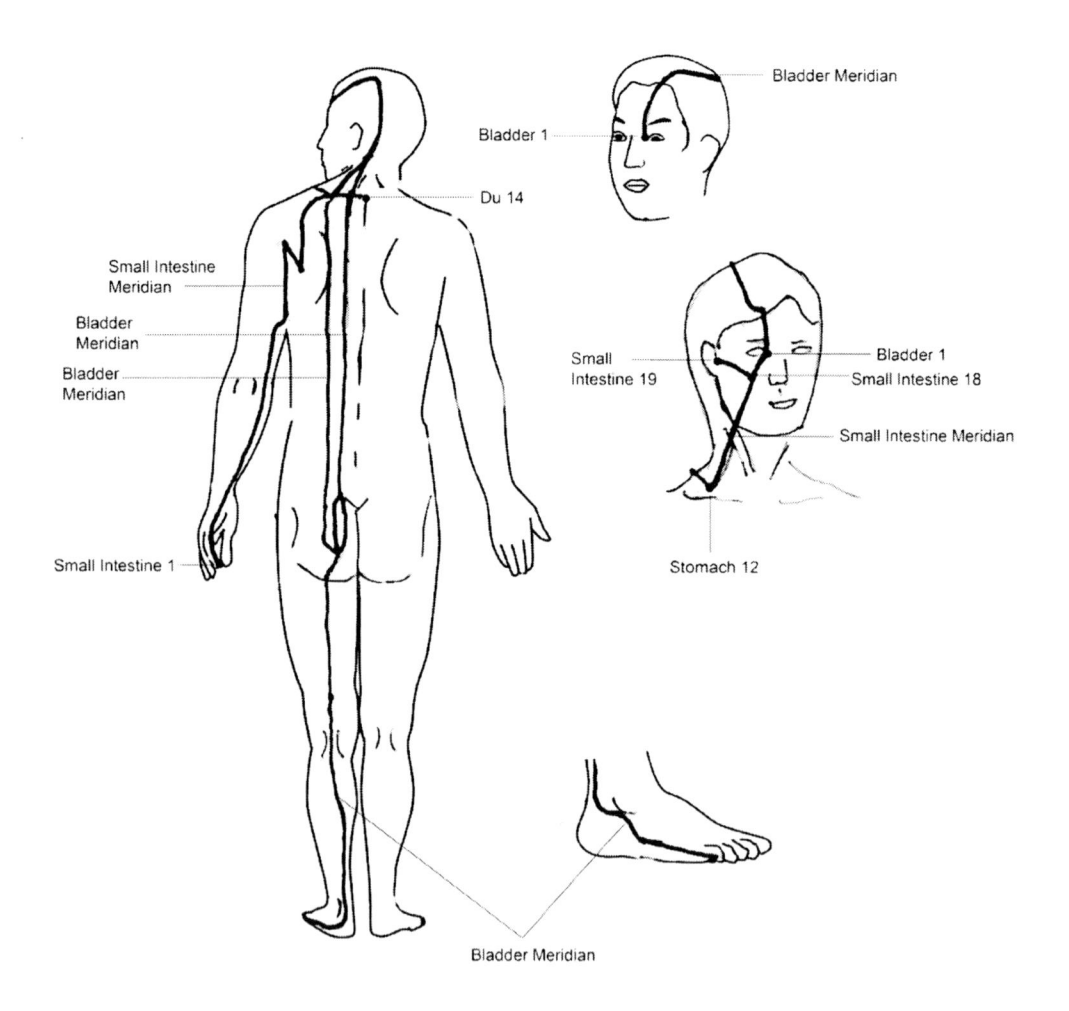

Hand & Foot Taiyang
(Small Intestine & Bladder Meridians)

Taiyang Channel

The Taiyang Channel is composed of the Small Intestine Channel of Hand Taiyang and the Bladder Channel of Foot Taiyang. The Taiyang channel covers the back, and back of the legs and arms. The Taiyang channel warms the exterior and moistens it. It protects the body from external pathogens by opening outward to send defensive (*wei*) qi to guard the surface layers of the body and to warm them in order to protect the body from cold. It can also close this area – like closing a gate – by closing the pores and contracting the muscles to prevent cold from invading. When you shiver, yang energy opening to the exterior is causing the muscles and surface tissues to contract in order to protect the exterior. To some degree, this warmth that spreads to the exterior relies on the Mingmen of the kidneys and the heart fire, hence the connection of Taiyang and Shaoyin. The *Huang Ti Nei Jing* describes disease of the Taiyang channel as follows:

> *The Taiyang channel takes charge of the superficies. When evil first invades man it is on the superficies, and when the evil and healthy energies contend, cold-heat will occur; if the evil stagnates between the muscle and the striae of the skin, carbuncle will occur. When the evil hurts the Foot-Taiyang bladder channel, the calf muscle where the channel passes will be come painful. The foot will also become flaccid and cold.*[48]

For Taiyang to be free from disease, yang qi and warmth must fill the outer body layers and move inward and outward appropriately. If Taiyang's movement is weak – excessively open – there can be sweating and fever. If its movement is excessively closed, yang qi can build up in the exterior causing body aches and impaired sweating, which prevents the expulsion of pathogenic qi.

---

[48] *Yellow Emperor's Canon of Internal Medicine*, Bing Wang, translated by Nelson Liansheng Wu and Andrew Qi Wu. China Science and Technology Press, p. 50.

Shaoyang

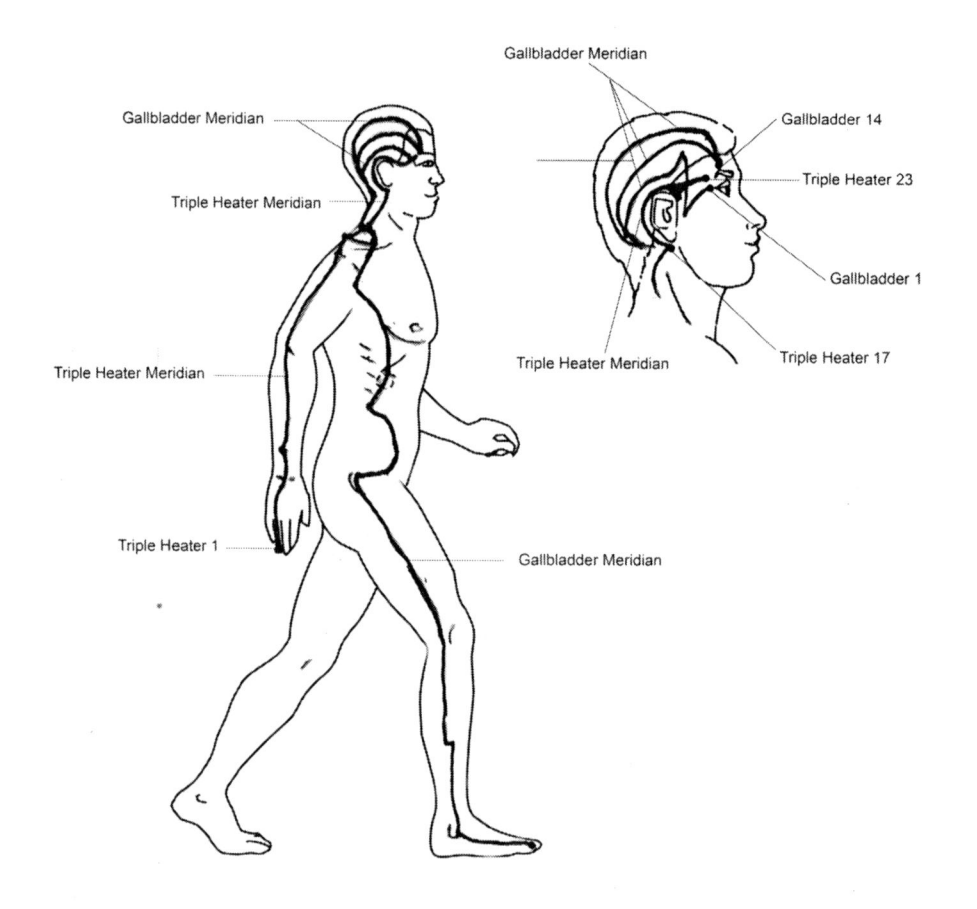

Hand and Foot Shaoyang
(Triple Heater & Gallbladder Meridians)

Shaoyang Channel

Shaoyang is composed of the Triple Heater Meridian[49] of Hand Shaoyang and the Gallbladder Meridian of Foot Shaoyang. Shaoyang energetically occupies a position that is half-interior and half-exterior. It is the hinge of open and close, therefore it regulates the movement of qi and blood between the interior and exterior. The internal pathways of the Triple Heater Meridian, in particular, carry Mingmen fire outward and return it to the interior. They also serve as pathways for fluid movement through the body. However, the Gallbladder also has a role in regulating qi and blood through its actions of overseeing and regulating digestive processes. Shaoyang also regulates movement in the spaces between the sinews and bones and has an association with the joints which are themselves a kind of pivot. In this way fluids are brought to the sinews and bones and metabolic waste is taken away.[50] For Shaoyang to operate correctly it must be free of blockage or stasis, so that communication is open between the interior and exterior. If Shaoyang pivots excessively, there can be a flaring up of fire and fluids causing sore throat and phlegm. If it does not pivot enough, fire from the interior - the Mingmen fire - cannot go outward and there may be cold extremities.[51]

---

[49] Often referred to as *San Jiao* or Triple Burner.
[50] *Applied Channel Theory in Chinese Medicine: Wang Ju-Yi's Lectures on Channel Therapeutics* by Wang Ju-Yi and Jason Robertson Seattle: Eastland Press, 2008, pp. 211-12.
[51] *Core Patterns of The Shang Han Lung: Part I.* Lecture by Arnaud Versluys. Pacific College of Oriental Medicine in NYC, 2009.

Yangming

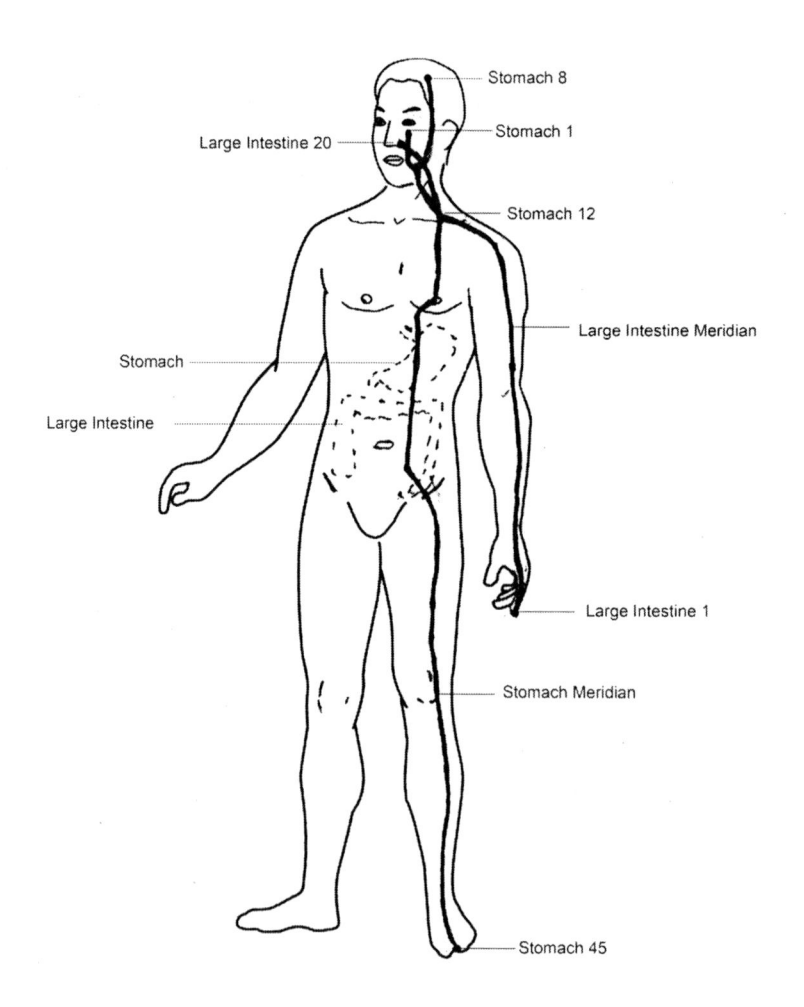

Hand and Foot Yangming
(Large Intestine & Stomach Meridians)

Yangming Channel

Yangming is composed of the Large Intestine Meridian of Hand Yangming and the Stomach Meridian of Foot Yangming. To some degree, Yangming can be understood to be the "Inside of the outside." Yangming is intimately involved with the processes of digestion through its connection with the stomach and large intestine. It regulates the movement of food and fluids through the pathways of digestion by fermenting and breaking down food and drink so that their nutrition and essence can be released inwardly. Therefore, Yangming closes or contracts toward the inside, directing the nutrients extracted from food and fluids inward toward the yin organs which transform this essence into blood, qi and body fluids. Because of this contracting and closing action, Yangming can be compared to a pressure cooker[52] which compresses qi inward toward the interior and the yin. Like a pressure cooker, Yangming needs heat (yang qi) to break down and "cook" food. Digestive processes must move smoothly toward the interior, otherwise the body will not be sufficiently supplied with qi and blood. If Yangming does not close properly, heat can build up in the exterior, causing high fever and thirst. If it closes too forcefully, digestive processes can stagnate, causing constipation, bloating (stagnant fluids), fullness and pain.[53]

---

[52] *Atlas of Acupuncture* by Claudia Focks. Churchill Livingstone (Elsevier Limited), 2008, p. 16.
[53] *Core Patterns of The Shang Han Lung: Part I.* Lecture by Arnaud Versluys. Pacific College of Oriental Medicine in NYC, 2009.

Taiyin

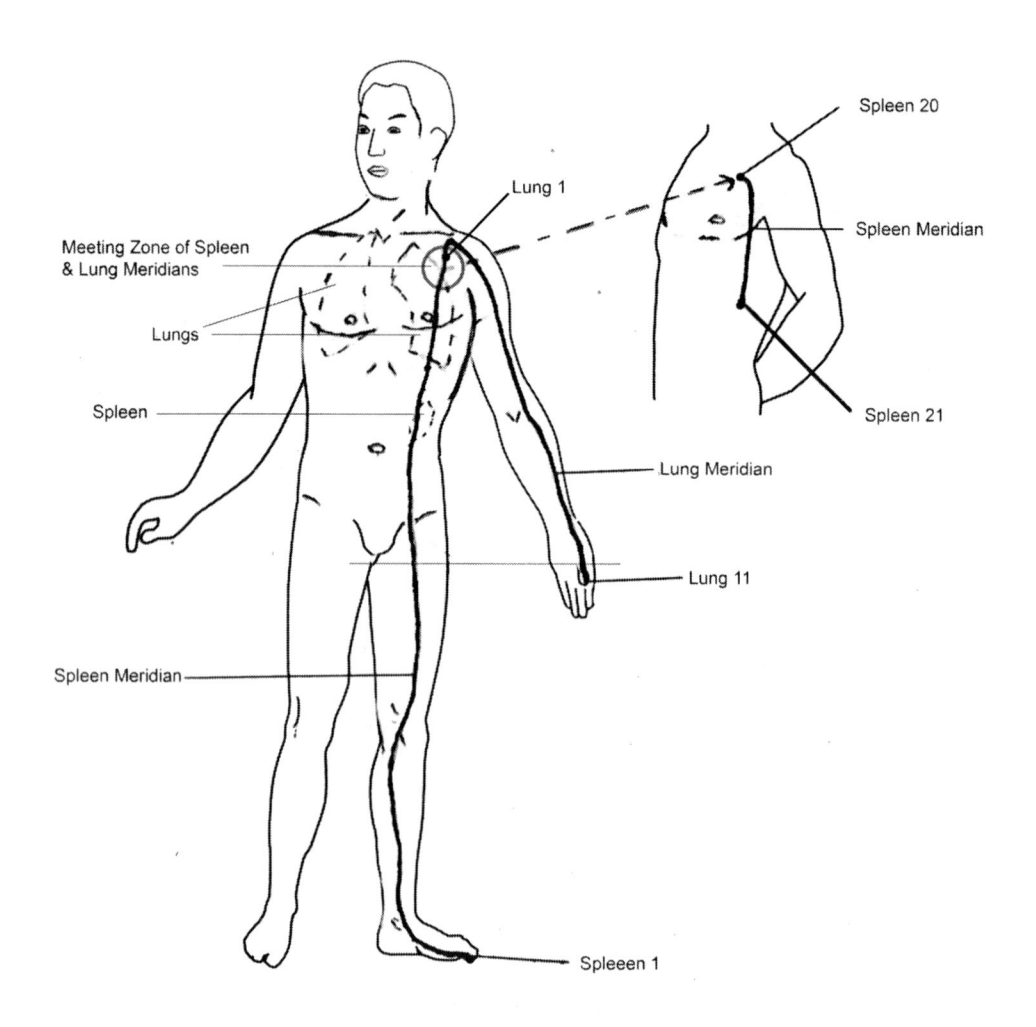

Hand and Foot Taiyin
(Lung and Spleen Meridians)

Taiyin Channel

Taiyin is composed of the Lung Meridian of Hand Taiyin and the Spleen Meridian of Foot Taiyin. Taiyin is the most superficial of the three yin. It can be thought of as the "outside of the inside," and is paired with Yangming. Like Taiyang, Taiyin is open, but whereas Taiyang opens to the outside, Taiyin opens to the internal organs. The post-natal qi derived from food and drink, which is broken down and processed by Yangming, is transformed into blood and refined fluids by Taiyin. Taiyin then opens inward, spreading these substances through the surrounding tissues to irrigate and to the nourish the organs and tissues. Taiyin is related to the spleen and lungs. The spleen disseminates fluids and nutrients throughout the body while the lungs disseminate the qi. If Taiyin opens too strongly, food and fluids are not properly transformed and there may be diarrhea, general fatigue and weakness and lack of appetite. If Taiyin does not open enough, the transformational aspect of digestion is impaired and there may be stagnation of fluids, bloating, water retention, abdominal fullness and cough.

Shaoyin

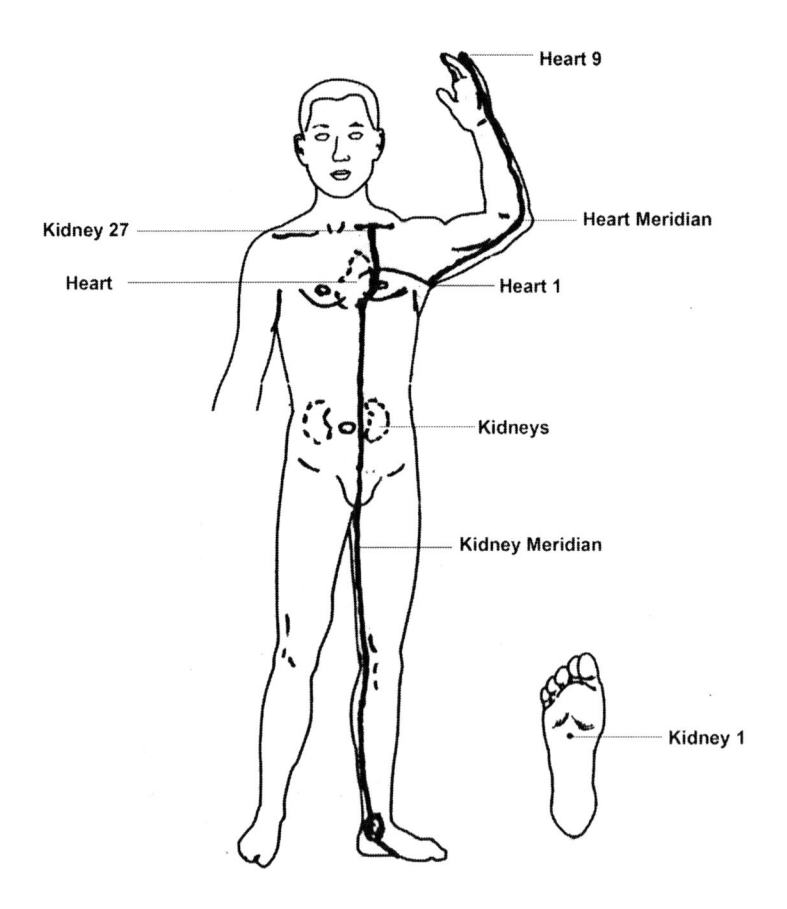

Hand and Foot Shaoyin
(Heart & Kidney Channels)

Shaoyin Channel

Shaoyin is composed of the Heart Meridian of Hand Shaoyin and the Kidney Meridian of Foot Shaoyin. Shaoyin is a hinge or a pivot between Taiyin and the inward gathering and closing of Jueyin. Shaoyin is related to the kidneys and the heart. Heart fire and the fire between the kidneys, *Mingmen,* circulate blood and fluids. In this sense, the Shaoyin pivot helps to regulate Taiyin, by aiding it in the dissemination of blood, fluids and qi. It also helps Jueyin by regulating the inward and outward movement of blood so that it can be stored and released properly by Jueyin.[54] Shaoyin is paired with Taiyang, which opens to the exterior. The body's heat is to some degree regulated by this connection. The Shaoyin pivot can move yang outward to warm the exterior or ventilate heat through sweating, or it can direct heat inward to warm the interior and activate circulation in the deeper levels of the body. If the Shaoyin pivot is weak, yang qi is not regulated properly and there may be sensations of heat and restlessness, and insomnia. If Shaoyin pivots and moves excessively, yang qi disperses and there may be fatigue, cold extremities, and drowsiness.[55]

---

[54] *Applied Channel Theory in Chinese Medicine: Wang Ju-Yi's Lectures on Channel Therapeutics* by Wang Ju-Yi and Jason Robertson Seattle: Eastland Press, 2008, p. 101.
[55] *Core Patterns of The Shang Han Lung: Part I.* Lecture by Arnaud Versluys. Pacific College of Oriental Medicine in NYC, 2009.

Jueyin

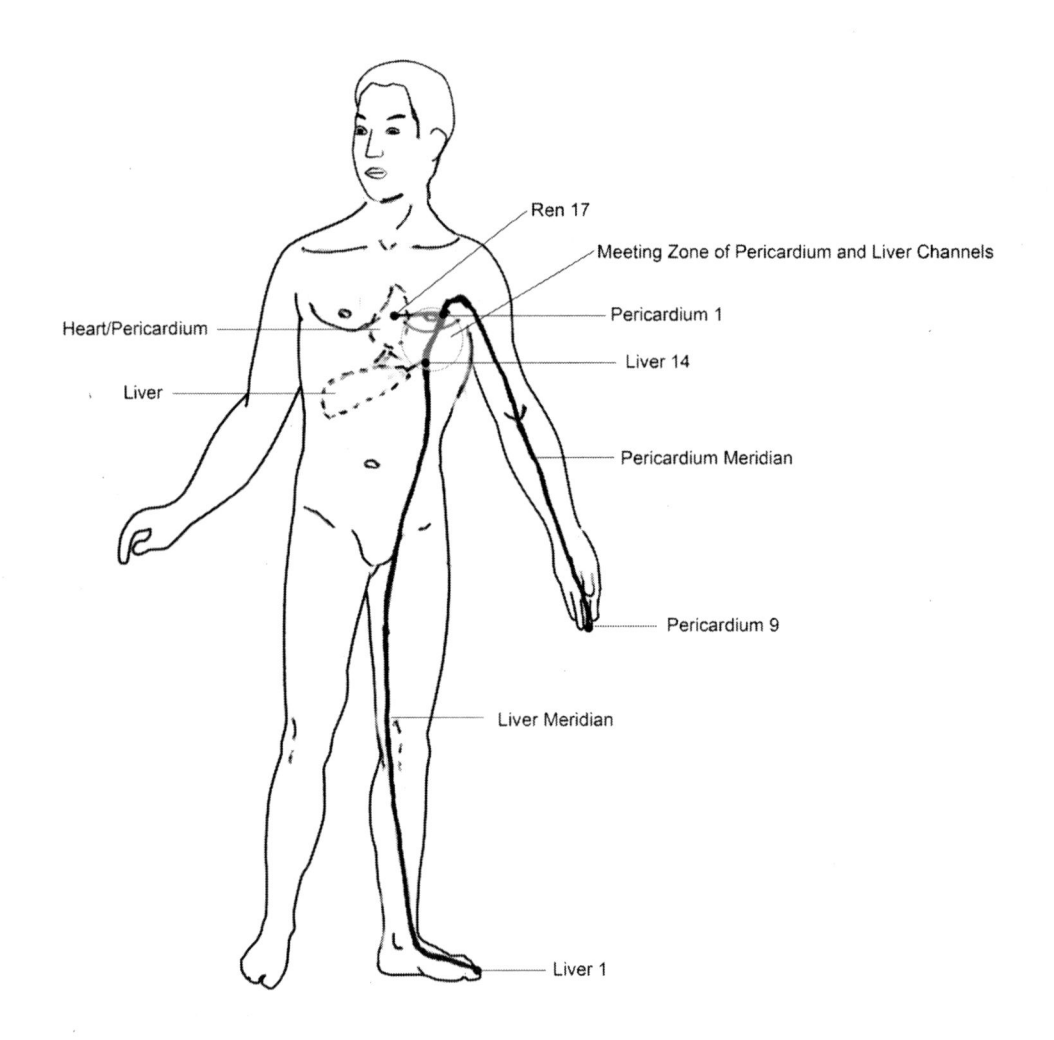

Hand and Foot Jueyin
(Pericardium and Liver Meridians)

Jueyin Channel

Jueyin is composed of the Pericardium Meridian of Hand Jueyin and the Liver Meridian of Foot Jueyin. Jueyin is the deepest of the yin axes. Jueyin is called "close" because it collects the yin energy (particularly blood) and transmits it to the interior of the body for storage and release. The liver stores the blood and releases it to the muscles and sinews during activity. The pericardium aids in this action as it is intimately connected with the heart and its role in circulating the blood. The pericardium protects the heart, not only because it is a double-walled sac that contains the heart, but also through its action of closing, which holds or contains the qi and emotions, releasing them outward at the appropriate time. When Jueyin closes excessively, there can be stasis of qi and or blood, qi stuck in the chest (chest pain or tightness) and cold extremities. If Jueyin does not close enough, there may be an upward surging of qi and heat.

Interaction of the 6 Yin-Yang Axes

Adapted from: Applied Channel Theory in Chinese Medicine: Wang Ju-Yi's Lectures on Channel Therapeutics by Wang Ju-Yi and Jason Robertson Seattle: Eastland Press, 2008, p. 253.

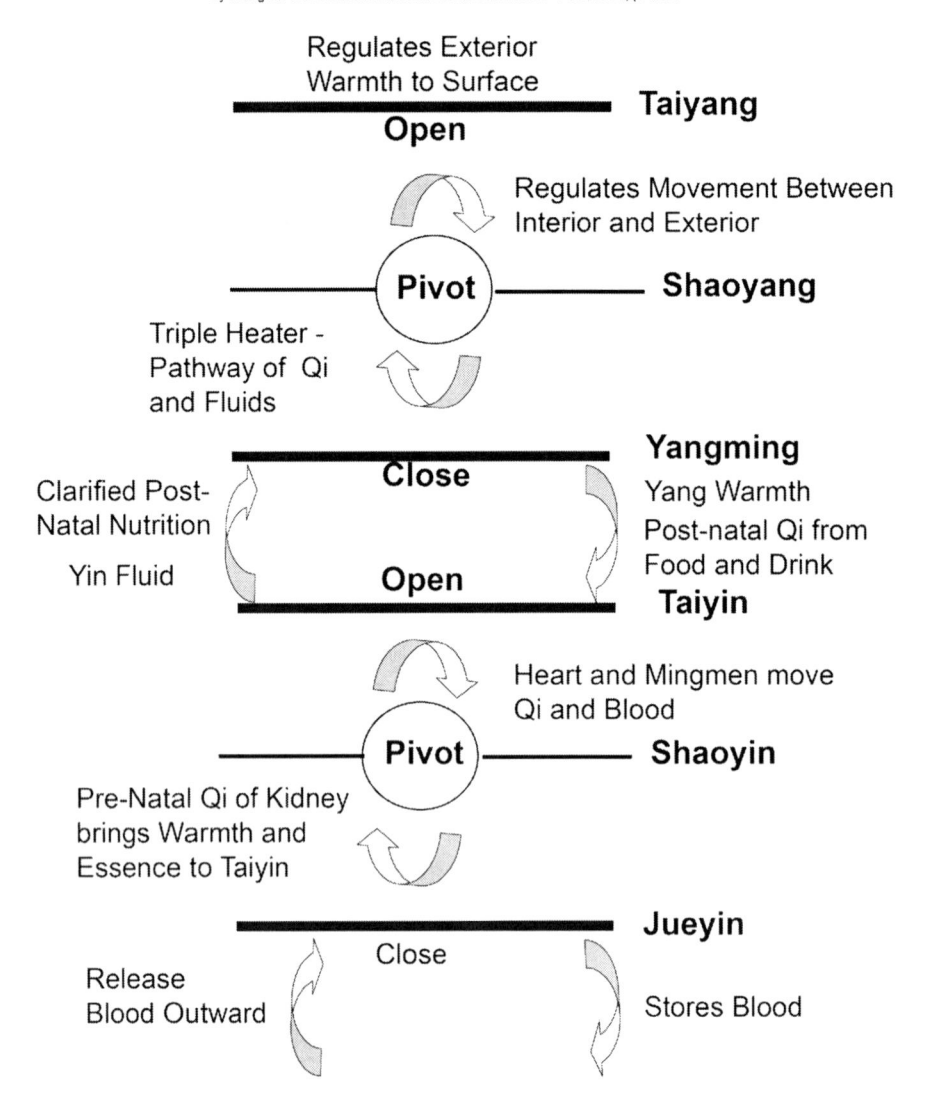

Taiyang — Open
Regulates Exterior Warmth to Surface

Shaoyang — Pivot
Regulates Movement Between Interior and Exterior
Triple Heater - Pathway of Qi and Fluids

Yangming — Close
Clarified Post-Natal Nutrition
Yin Fluid
Yang Warmth
Post-natal Qi from Food and Drink

Taiyin — Open

Shaoyin — Pivot
Heart and Mingmen move Qi and Blood
Pre-Natal Qi of Kidney brings Warmth and Essence to Taiyin

Jueyin — Close
Release Blood Outward
Stores Blood

Five Phases and Six Axes

To thoroughly understand the Six Axes, one should be familiar with Five Phase (Five Element) Theory and the functions of the Zang Fu (the internal organs). The next section outlines the primary functions of the organs according to traditional Chinese medicine. This book is not the place for an exhaustive discussion of their functions and interactions. It is important to keep in mind that although the organs are physical entities they are defined by their energetic functions and inter-relationships which are themselves expressions of yin qi and yang qi. The meridian pathways, the movement of qi and other substances along those pathways, and the organ functions are therefore interwoven and inseparable.

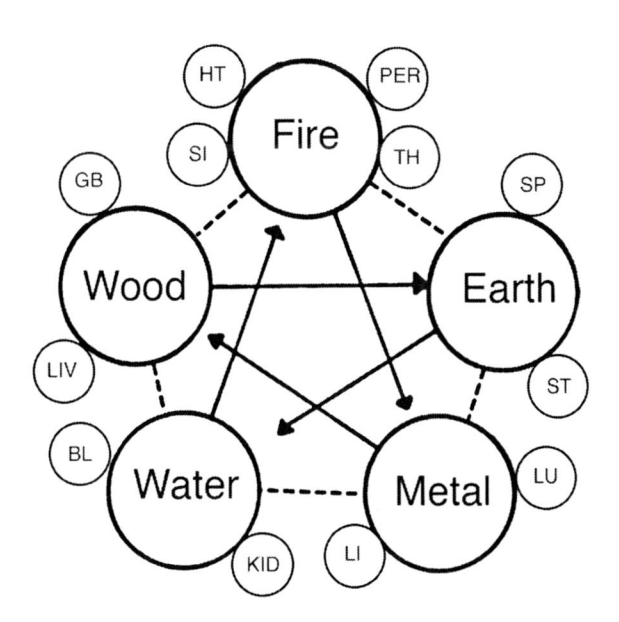

The Five Phases and Associated Organs

Jueyin: Pericarium and Liver
Shaoyang: Triple Heater and Gallbladder
Storage and release of Qi and
Blood to the tissues and organs

Shao-yang (pivot)
Jueyin (close)

Shaoyin (pivot)
Taiyang (open)

Taiyin (open)
Yangming (close)

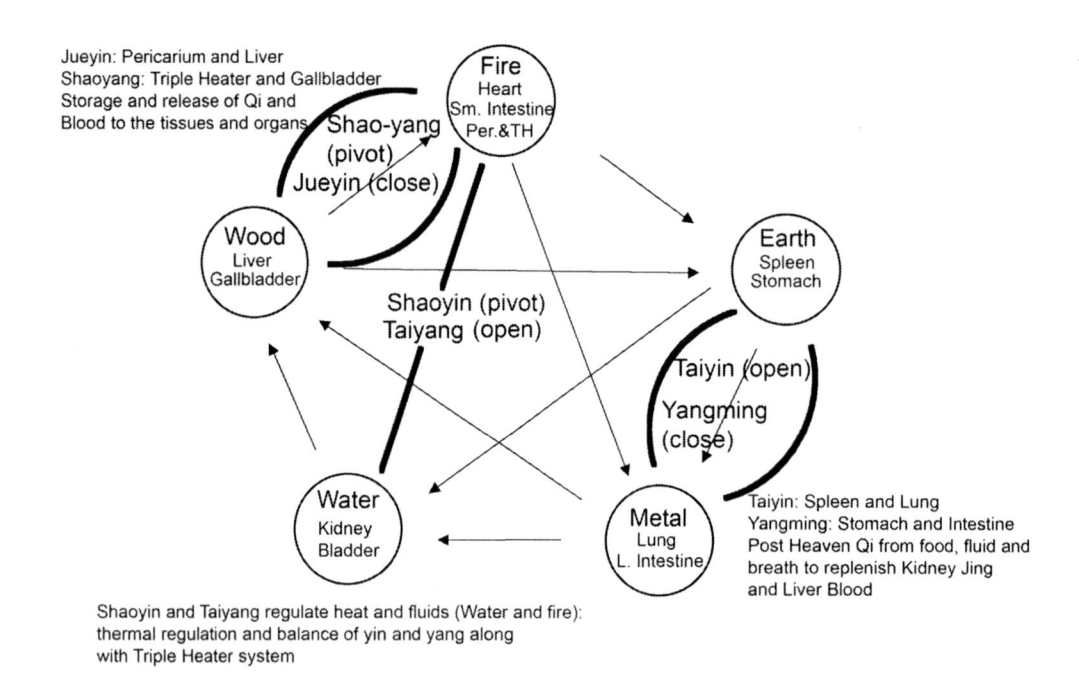

Fire — Heart, Sm. Intestine, Per.&TH

Wood — Liver, Gallbladder

Earth — Spleen, Stomach

Water — Kidney, Bladder

Metal — Lung, L. Intestine

Taiyin: Spleen and Lung
Yangming: Stomach and Intestine
Post Heaven Qi from food, fluid and breath to replenish Kidney Jing and Liver Blood

Shaoyin and Taiyang regulate heat and fluids (Water and fire): thermal regulation and balance of yin and yang along with Triple Heater system

**Five Phase Relationships of the Six Divisions:
The Three Yin and Three Yang Axes**

The First Energetic Unit: Taiyin & Yangming

Taiyin is the Lung and Spleen

Yangming is Large Intestine and Stomach

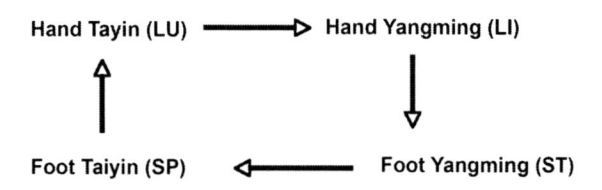

```
Hand Taiyin (LU) ─────▷ Hand Yangming (LI)
      ▲                        │
      │                        ▼
Foot Taiyin (SP) ◁───── Foot Yangming (ST)
```

Spleen and Stomach are Earth: earth generates metal and controls water. Lung and Large Intestine are Metal: metal generates water and controls wood.

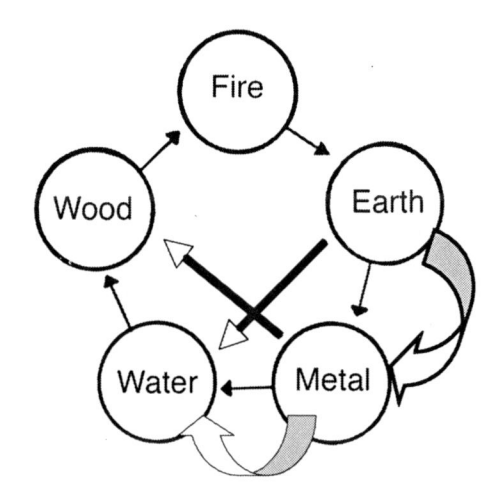

SPLEEN (*PI*)

The Spleen Governs Transportation (*yun*) and Transformation (*hua*)

The Spleen Governs (controls) the Blood

The Spleen Controls the Raising of the Qi and Holds Up the Organs

The Spleen Controls the Muscles/Flesh and the 4 Limbs

The Spleen Opens into the Mouth

The Spleen Manifests in the Lips

The Spleen is the Residence of the *Yi* (thought)

The Spleen Loathes Dampness

LUNGS (*FEI*)

The Lungs Rule the Qi & Govern Respiration

The Lungs Control the Channels and the Blood Vessels

The Lungs Control Descending & Dispersing

The Lungs Regulate (move & direct) the Water Passages

The Lungs Open into the Nose

The Lungs Govern the Voice

The Lungs Loathe Dryness

The Lungs House the *Po* (corporeal soul)

STOMACH (*WEI*)

The Stomach Controls the Rotting & Ripening of Food

The Stomach Controls Descending

The Stomach is the Source of the 12 Channels and the Sea of Water and Grains

The Stomach Dislikes Dryness & Likes Dampness

LARGE INTESTINE (*DA CHANG*)

The Large Intestine Connects with the Small Intestine and the Anus.

The Large intestine receives the Turbid from the Small Intestine and Separates the Clear from the Turbid. (Clear goes to kidneys; Turbid is Expelled)

The Second Energetic Unit: Shaoyin & Taiyang

Shaoyin is Heart and Kidneys

Taiyang is Small Intestine and Bladder

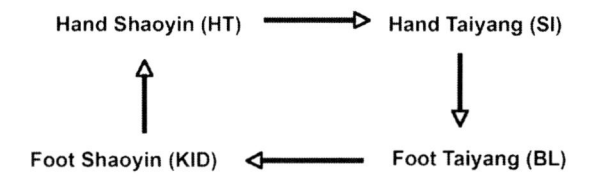

```
Hand Shaoyin (HT)  ———▷  Hand Taiyang (SI)
       △                         │
       │                         ▽
Foot Shaoyin (KID) ◁———   Foot Taiyang (BL)
```

Kidneys and Bladder are Water: water generates wood and controls fire

Heart and Small Intestine are Fire: fire generates earth and controls metal.

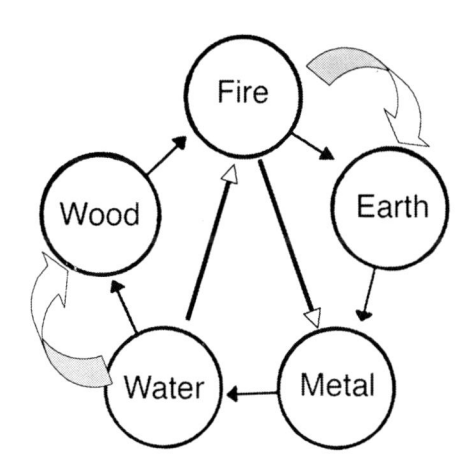

HEART (*XIN*)

The Heart Rules the Blood

The Heart Controls the Blood Vessels

The Heart Houses the *Shen* (spirit)

The Heart Manifests in the Complexion

The Heart Opens into the Tongue

The Heart Loathes Heat

Sweat is the Fluid of the Heart

KIDNEYS (SHEN)

The Kidneys Store the *Jing* (essence)

The Kidneys are the Root of Yin and Yang and the Source of Fire and Water

The Kidneys Control Growth, Development and Reproduction

The Kidneys Rule the Bones

The Kidneys Govern Water

The Kidneys Control the Reception of Qi

The Kidneys Control the Lower Orifices

The Kidneys Open Into the Ear

The Kidneys Manifest in the Hair (on the head)

The Kidneys Loathe The Cold

The Kidneys House the *Zhi* (will)

SMALL INTESTINE (XIAO CHANG)

The Small Intestine Receives, Controls and Absorbs

The Small Intestine Separates the Pure From the Impure (The Clear From the Tubid)

The Small Intestine Separates Fluids

BLADDER (PANG GUANG)

The Bladder Stores and Excretes Urine

The Third Energetic Unit: Jueyin & Shaoyang

Jueyin is Pericardium and Liver

Shaoyang is Triple Heater and Gallbladder

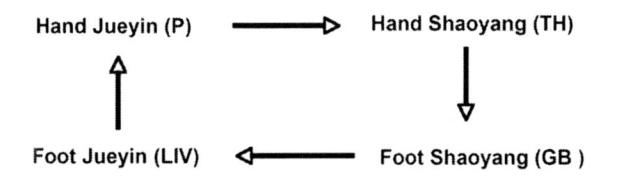

```
Hand Jueyin (P)  ────────▷  Hand Shaoyang (TH)
      ▲                              │
      │                              ▼
Foot Jueyin (LIV) ◁──────── Foot Shaoyang (GB)
```

Pericardium and Triple Heater are Fire: fire generates earth and controls metal.

Liver and Gallbladder are Wood: wood generates fire and controls earth.

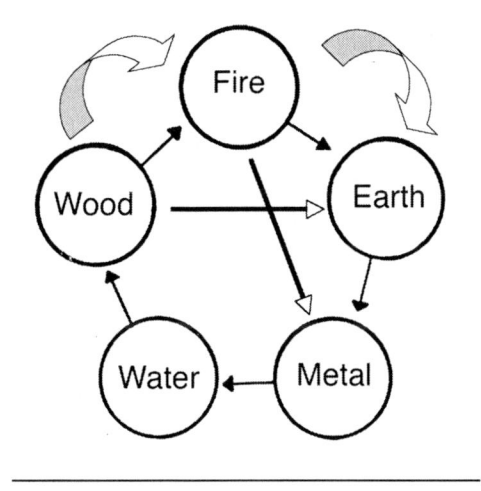

LIVER (*GAN*)

The Liver Stores the Blood

The Liver Ensures the Smooth Flow of Qi Throughout the Body

The Liver Controls the Sinews (*jin*)

The Liver Manifests in the Nails

The Liver Opens Into the Eyes

The Liver is the Residence of the Hun (Ethereal Soul)

The Liver is in Charge of Strategy and Planning

The Liver Loathes Wind

PERICARDIUM (XIN BAO)

The Pericardium Protects the Heart

The Pericardium is The Envoy of Heart

GALLBLADDER (DAN)

The Gallbladder Stores & Secretes Bile

The Gallbladder is Responsible for Decision Making and Courage

TRIPLE HEATER (SAN JIAO)

The Water Pathways Issue From the Triple Heater

The Triple Heater Disseminates the Original Qi (yuan qi)

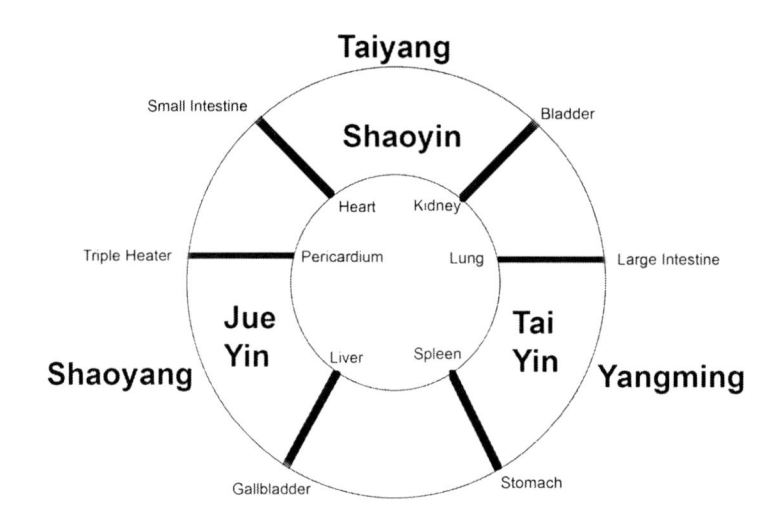

Circular Model - Relationship of Five Elements and Six Axes

(adapted from Acupuncture Energetice by Joseph Helms, p. 222-3)

The Eight Trigrams and the Five Elements

Ba Gua traditionally uses the eight trigrams as the basis of its theory. The Ding Shi palms are thought by some to have a relationship to the eight trigrams and the sixty-four hexagrams of the *Yi Jing* (I Ching). Likewise the Eight Extraordinary meridians are often thought to be related to the Eight Trigrams. In practice many practitioners use Five Phase theory to explain Ba Gua's health promoting aspect. King Wen's post-heaven arrangement of the Eight Trigrams makes this possible as the Five Phases are themselves an expression of the Post-Heaven (Post-Natal) energies that move within us and within the world around us. As we shall see in later chapters, the Extraordinary Meridians are thought to be an expression of the Pre-Heaven (Pre-Natal) energies that move and interact within us. The following diagram illustrates the relationship of the post-heaven trigrams and their manifestation in the Five Phases.

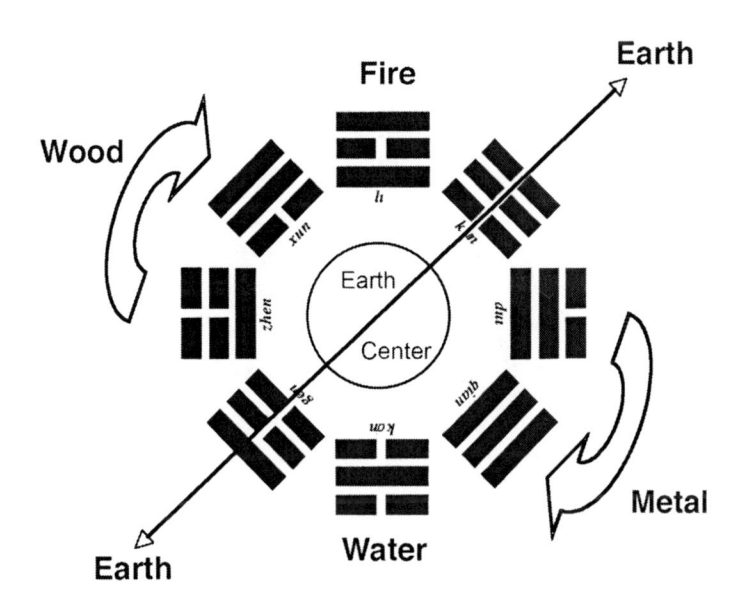

Five Elements and Eight Trigrams

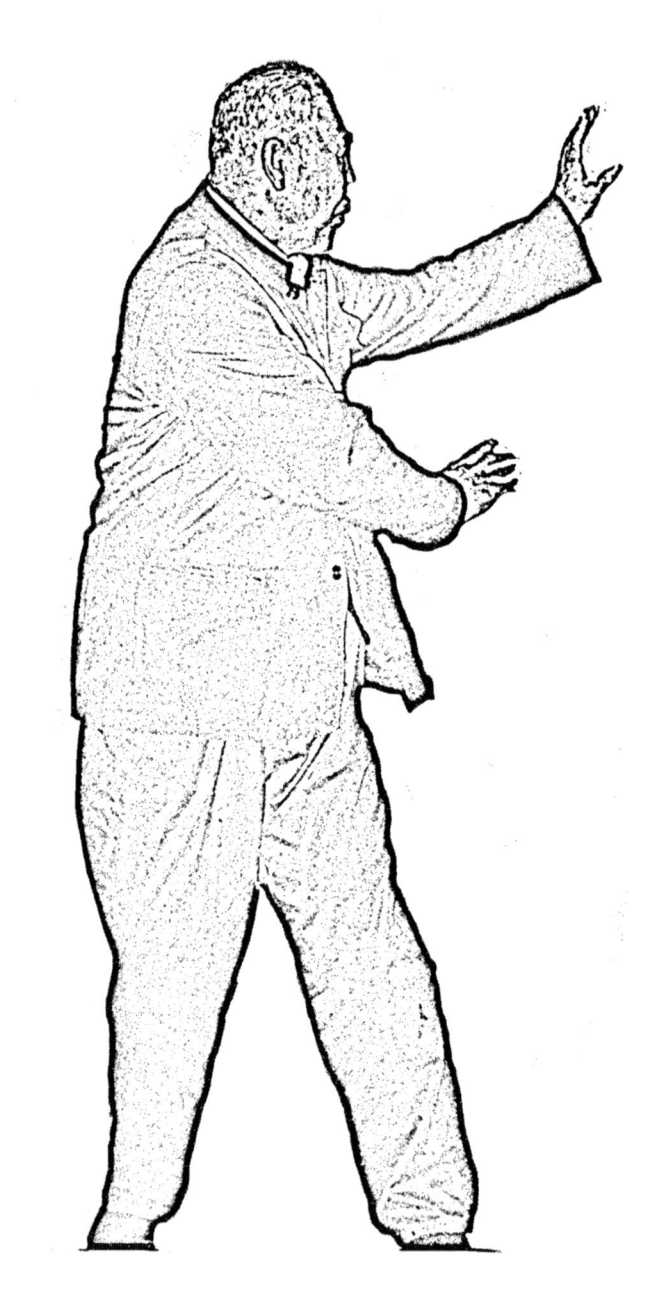

Millstone Pushing Palm
From an author photo of Wang Shi Tong

Chapter 8
The Eight Extraordinary Channels

The Eight Extraordinary Channels - *Qi Jing Ba Mai*

The *Qi Jing Ba Mai* or Eight Extraordinary Vessels have been the subject of much debate in Chinese medicine. Although modern medical texts show these meridians as having discrete pathways, there is a recognition that they are not so much pathways as a kind of matrix of energetic organization that balances, supplements and harmonizes the activities of the three yin and three yang axes discussed in the previous chapter. In Nei Gong practices and the Daoist tradition of meditation and internal alchemy, descriptions of the extraordinary vessels are often different than those in the medical texts. This has led to some confusion in conceptualizing the energetic trajectories of these channels. Many modern authors believe that the energetic matrix represented by Eight Extraordinary Vessels begins to develop at conception and continues to form throughout the various stages of fetal development.[56] There is speculation that the Mingmen ("life gate"), also known as the "moving qi between the kidneys," comes into being at conception and has an association with Chong Mai (The Thrusting Channel). Ren Mai and Du Mai originate from the "moving qi" and represent the basic division of yin and yang in the body - Du Mai rising up the back of the body and Ren Mai descending down the front.

> *Heaven and Earth have noon and midnight, the body has Ren Mai and Du Mai as its polar axes. The Du Mai, Ren Mai and Chong Mai have different names, but in the end they are the same and have the same significance. The Chong Mai insures the inseparability of the Ren Mai and Du Mai – of yin and yang. If we tried to separate yin*

---

[56] *Acupuncture Energetics: A Clinical Approach for Physicians,* by Joseph M. Helms, Berkely CA: Medical Acupuncture Publishers, 1995, p. 523.

and yang, we would have to realize hat they are an "inseparable whole," a unit.[57]

The extraordinary meridians are called *qi* 奇 ("marvelous; strange; rare; extraordinary"). They are both *Mai* (vessels) and *Jing* (meridians). They are named in relation to the twelve primary meridians which are called the *Jing Zheng. Zheng* (正) means "straight; right; correct; ordinary; without any diversion." The unusual nature of the Eight Extraordinary Vessels stems from their differences from the Twelve Primary Meridians. Unlike the primary meridians, the Eight Extraordinary Vessels:

1. Have no hand or foot designation.
2. Are not necessarily divided into yin or yang pairs.
3. Have no specific, primary connection to the internal organs (*Zang Fu*).
4. Relate to the Five Elements or Five Phases in an indirect rather than a direct way.
5. Aside form the Ren and Du channels, do not have their own acupoints.
6. Are not connected directly with the three yin and three yang energetic axes, but instead connect, supplement and balance these axes.[58]

---

[57] *Atlas of Acupuncture* by Claudia Focks. Churchill Livingstone (Elsevier Limited), 2008, p. 24.
[58] *The Eight Extraordinary Meridians,* by Claude Larre and Eisabeth Rochat de la Vallee. Monkey Press 1997, pp. 6-8.

General Functions of The Eight Extraordinary Vessels

The Eight Extraordinary Vessels are believed to circulate *Jing* (essence) and *Yuan Qi* ("source qi"; "original qi"), which are the transmitters of life and provide the energetic and physical substrate that both nourishes and formulates the energetic matrix of the body. In this regard, one of the important functions of the Eight Extraordinary Vessels is to circulate and transport *Yuan Qi* and *Jing* to and from the primary meridians and the various tissues of the body. Other general functions include:

1. The Eight Extraordinary Vessels act as lakes and reservoirs which store qi, blood, yin and yang, releasing these energies into the primary meridians when they are needed. In this role they can absorb any overflow of qi from the primary meridians and their collateral vessels and redistribute this overflow elsewhere.

2. The Eight Extraordinary Vessels help to maintain the cohesion and proper functioning of the primary channels. In this sense they help to integrate and connect the six yin-yang energetic axes.

3. The Eight Extraordinary Vessels circulate *Wei Qi* (defensive energy) to the exterior of the body particularly in the thorax, abdomen and back.

4. The Eight Extraordinary Vessels circulate and carry out functions that are outside the scope of the primary Jing Luo system.

Nei Gong and The Extraordinary Vessels

In Nei Gong and Daoist internal alchemy, The Eight Extraordinary Vessels are often referred to as the "Eight Psychic Channels." This name is attributed to the Extraordinary Vessels because of their connection to the deepest energetic levels of a individual's being. Therefore, they are regarded by some sources as having a connection to that person's fundamental "personality" or "character." In the context of meditation, internal alchemy, martial arts and Nei Gong practices, the Eight Extraordinary Vessels have two important functions. When they are free from obstruction, they:

1. Allow for the *Jing Qi*, the vital generative force of the kidneys to move and transform freely.
2. Allow the qi and the breath to flow unimpeded through all the channels, meridians and interstices of the body.

Opening the Eight Extraordinary Vessels is therefore a key part of converting generative force to spirit in meditation and Nei Gong in order to preserve the health of the body and resist disease.

The nucleus of the Eight Extraordinary Vessels consists of four channels. These four channels are interlinked and act in a unified fashion to circulate the Jing Qi. They orient the vertical, horizontal, front and back, and center lines of the body.

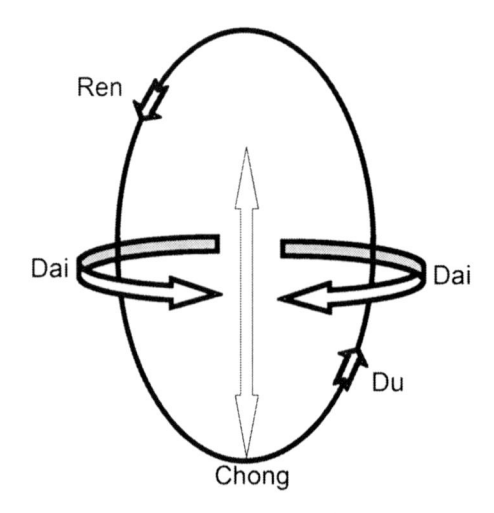

Orientation of the Four Central Extra Vessels:
Ren, Du, Chong and Dai Vessels

1. Du Mai (Governing or Directing Vessel) rises from the perineum through the spine and enters the brain at the nape. Then it continues up and over the head and connects with Ren Mai in the mouth.

2. Ren Mai (Control or Conception Vessel) joins with Du Mai in the brain and mouth and then descends down the front of the body to the pubic bone and the genital organs where it again connects with Du Mai creating a circuit.

3. Chong Mai (Thrusting or Penetrating Vessel) runs up the center of the body. When connected and flowing freely, Ren Mai, Du Mai and Chong Mai are sometimes referred to as a single entity: The Central Channel.

4. Dai Mai (Belt or Girdle Vessel) is like a girdle around the area of the Dan Tian and kidneys that both connects with and wraps the Ren and Du channels and all of the other meridians of the body. Unlike the other meridians which primarily run longitudinally through the body, Dai Mai runs horizontally around the body at the level of the waist.

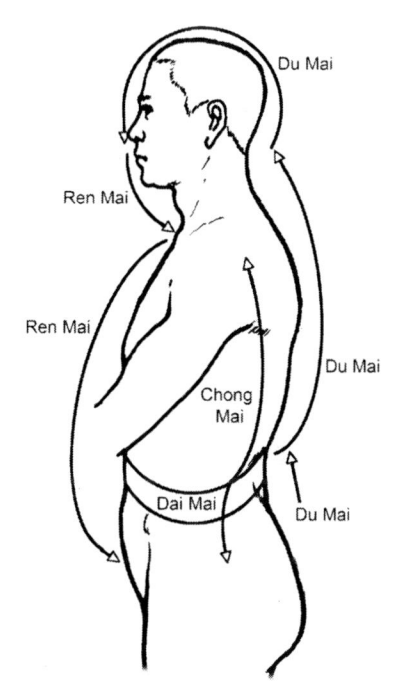

The Four Central Extra Channels

The Micro-Cosmic Orbit and The Extraordinary Vessels

Medical texts show Ren Mai traveling upwards from the genitals to the chin and face, but in Daoist meditation and Nei Gong, Du Mai and Ren Mai form a circuit in which breath, qi, and generative force (essence or *Jing*) flow upward along the Du channel and downward along the Ren. This circulation is called the Small Heavenly Circulation (*Xiao Zhou Tian*) or Micro-Cosmic Orbit. In this context the two vertical channels (Du and Ren) cut across the Belt Channel (Dai Mai) linking it with the heart above and the generative gate (genitals) below, with the navel in front, and the kidneys behind and the thrusting Channel (Chong Mai) in the center of the body. The other four channels - Yin Qiao Mai, Yang Qiao Mai, Yin Wei Mai and Yang Wei Mai - circulate the Jing Qi from the soles of the feet to the shoulders and head, from the shoulders to the hands and from the hands back to the chest.[59]

Modern medical texts show these four vessels as originating in the feet and ascending upward to the head, without passing into the upper limbs, while Nei Gong and alchemical texts often describe them as follows:

The **Yang Wei Mai (Yang Linking Vessels)** in the outer sides of both arms link the shoulders with the palm centers after passing through the middle fingers.

The **Yin Wei (Yin Linking Vessels)** in the inner sides of the two arms link the palm centers with the chest.

The **Yang Qiao Mai (Yang Heel Vessels)** rise from the centers of the soles of the feet and heel and turn along the outside of the ankles and legs to reach the base of the penis (ie: the genitals) where they connect other channels.

---

[59] *Taoist Yoga: Alchemy & Immortality* by Lu K'uan Yu (Charles Luk). Maine: Samuel Weiser, Inc. 1973, pp. 22-3.

The **Yin Qiao Mai (Yin Heel Vessels)** rise from the sole and the heels and turn along the inside of the ankles and legs before reaching the base of the penis where they connect other channels.[60]

In the practice of Daoist alchemy, one of the first steps in is to clear the Eight Psychic Channels of blockage, thereby opening and purifying them before going on to other stages of the practice. This is sometimes called the *Da Zhou Tian* – Large Heavenly Circulation or Macro-Cosmic Orbit. Five breaths are employed to circulate the breath and vital force through the eight channels:

First Breath:
- Inhale and let the qi and breath rise up Du Mai to enter the brain.
- Exhale and let the qi and breath descend down Ren Mai to return to Dan Tian and the genitals.

Second Breath:
- Inhale and let the qi and breath go up the navel via Ren Mai and enter the Dai Mai to go to the back and rise up either side of the spine to reach the shoulders.
- Exhale and let the qi and breath flow from the shoulders down the Yang Wei channels on the outside of the arms to the middle fingers and then to the palm centers.

Third Breath:
- Inhale and let the qi and breath return to the chest by flowing through the Yin Wei channels on the inside of the arms.
- Exhale and let the qi and breath return to the belt channel where the two branches reunite before returning to Dan Tian.

---

[60] Ibid, p. 21.

Fourth Breath:
- Inhale and let the qi and breath rise through the Chong Mai to the area of the solar plexus under the heart where it stops. "On no account should it rise above the heart."
- Exhale and let the qi and breath return to the Dantian and then from there divide and flow down the outer sides of the legs and ankles through Yang Qiao Mai to reach the bubbling well points (Yong Quan) on the soles of the feet

Fifth Breath:
- Inhale and let the qi and breath flow into the Yin Qiao Channels to rise from the soles up the inner sides of the knees and ankles to return to the Dantian.
- Exhale and let the qi and breath return to the genitals.[61]

One Qi and One Breath

It should be understood that these five breaths are merely a means to begin to conceptualize the circulation of vital force – qi and breath - in the Eight Extraordinary Channels. Ultimately, there is one qi in the body and one breath. Rather then qi and breath circulating sequentially through these vessels, the rising and falling, ascent and descent, outward movement and inward movement, all take place simultaneously. Like the spokes of a wheel, or the paddles on a waterwheel, as one rises, one falls; as something goes outward, something moves inward. In the same way, although in the medical texts and even in the Nei Gong texts the flow of vital force in the channels is described as having a direction, in fact, vital force flows in both

---
[61] Ibid, pp. 24-5.

directions through the primary meridians and the extraordinary vessels. Hence it is said:

> *In one pathway [of qi] the breath of Heaven and Earth, the Jingqi is accepted into Dantian while the Zhenqi [True Qi] in the Dantian is transported from the armpits to the vertex. While this ascending occurs, the Zhenqi is also descending from Yu Kou [an area behind the heart] to Dantian. This is one qi arising from origin. From the Dantian, Zhenqi is transported downward from the crotch to the Dantian at the sole of the foot. As qi goes downward, there is simultaneous rising from the sole, up the lateral side of the thigh to Dantian. Left and right together make two qi arising from the origin. From the Dantian Zhenqi is transported to the back, from whence the qi again descends returning to Dantian. Left and right together make two qi arising from the origin. All together five qi arise from the origin. One ascends and one descends; one falls, one rises; one goes out, one enters in; without contradiction; flowing constantly, without stopping, without end.*[62]

The common element in different Nei Gong practices is the circulation of breath and qi up the Du channel and down the Ren Channel. Within these two vessels the primordial qi is engendered and the "true breath" arises. Because these two channels have a single source at the Mingmen and organs of reproduction, they are considered to be expressions of the primordial yin and yang energies of the body. Once they are fully open to the circulation of qi and breath, "the hundred meridians open" naturally and spontaneously. In Ba Gua Circle Walking Nei Gong, the first

---

[62] *Nei Gong: The Authentic Classic – A Translation of the Nei Gong Zhen Chuan,* translated by Tom Bisio, Huang Guo-Qi and Joshua Paynter. Outskirts Press Inc, 2011, pp. 20-21.

palm position - Downward Sinking Palm - in combination with the rotation of the body and the turning of the steps around the circle, stimulates and opens the circulation the Ren and Du vessels. By extension the Chong vessel, which lies between Ren and Du and pulses qi between the heart and kidneys, also opens.

The famous Ming dynasty physician Li Shi Zhen stressed the relationship between Daoist meditation, Nei Gong practices and the Extraordinary Vessels. In these practices the cultivation of internal stillness and emptiness is the basis from which the primordial yang moves to activate and open these vessels, particularly Chong Mai, Ren Mai and Du Mai. However the other Extraordinary Vessels are also important in the cultivation of internal emptiness:

> *It is dependant on the other extraordinary vessels in various ways. The Wei vessels define the structural and energetic boundaries for this process of energetic refinement. The Yin Qiao vessel connects the extraordinary vessels with the macrocosmic expression of the primal yang. The Dai vessel regulates all of the other extraordinary vessels.*[63]

DU MAI (Governing Vessel)

Du (督) means to "superintend" "govern" "regulate" or "direct." Du can also mean, "the controller." It refers to the governor of a province or the commander in chief of the armed forces in an area. *The Du may be understood in militaristic and political terms as an allusion to the imperial title of Director General (Zong Du 總督), a term in use since the Former Han, denoting one who is generally in charge, typically of regional clusters*

---

[63] *An Exposition of the Extraordinary Vessels: Acupuncture, Alchemy & Internal Medicine* by Charles Chace and Miki Shima. Seattle: Eastland Press, 2010, p. 65.

of two or more provinces.[64]. Du can also mean "the capital," and is therefore considered to be the capital of the yang vessels. The Du vessel regulates all the yang channels in the body. Du also refers to being upright and centered - *Zheng Zong* (正中)[65] - a reference to the central channel.

Zhuang Zi (Chuang Tzu) refers to the Du channel as the "central meridian," whose flowing current is unseen, the real controller of life in opposition to the conscious mind's pretensions of control.[66] In this context, the Du is considered to be central and to remain still - *leaning neither left nor right, occupying the position of a channel of energy but without palpable physical form. To follow along the Du is to proceed along the empty channel with a clear, weightless, subtle energy, halting whenever one cannot further proceed. This flow is naturally smooth, for it always finds the center.*[67]

Du Mai commands the yang of the body. Du Mai regulates all of the yang channels in the body. It is the "Sea of Yang Vessels." The master point of Du Mai is Huo Xi ("Back Ravine") – SI 3. Du Mai and Taiyang are connected in several places and the small intestine, the yang organ of the fire element, has a connection with *Mingmen* (the moving qi between the kidneys), the yang of water.

---

[64] *Applied Channel Theory in Chinese Medicine: Wang Ju-Yi's Lectures on Applied Channel Therapeutics* by Wang Ju-Yi and Jason D. Robertson. Seattle: Eastland Press, 2008, p. 289.
[65] Ibid.
[66] *Zhuangzi: The Essential Writings with Selections from Traditional Commentaries.* Translated by Brooke Ziporyn. Indianapolis and Cambridge: Hackett Publishing Co. Inc, 2009, pp.21-2.
[67] Ibid, Commentary by Wang Fuzhi, p. 167.

Master Point:
Du Mai

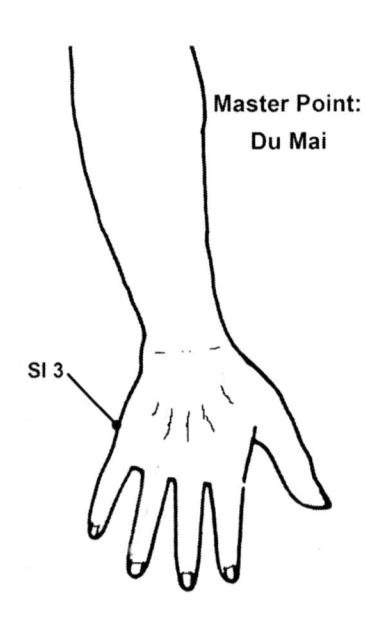

SI 3

Du Mai is intimately involved with the posture. If the back is not straight and aligned, then the flow of qi through the Du channel will not be optimal. In turn, this will weaken the Ren Channel as these two channels operate as a unified circuit. Because the Du and Ren Vessels are central and integral to the functioning of the other channels, poor posture can weaken the entire meridian system and negatively impact body, mind and spirit. Hence the importance of correct posture in the practice of Nei Gong and martial arts.

Du Mai Functions, Connections & Associations

- Du Mai has an ascending movement.
- Du Mai rises up the back to connect with the brain.
- Du Mai emanates from the *Mingmen*, kidneys and genitals and emerges at the *Huiyin* acu-point (Ren 1 in the perineum).
- Du Mai has a connection with the *Jing* (essence) and the yin of the kidneys.

- Du Mai has a direct relationship with the spine and brain (the "Sea of Marrow"). The brain is filled with marrow - modern authors often interpret cerebrospinal fluid as being a component of brain marrow.

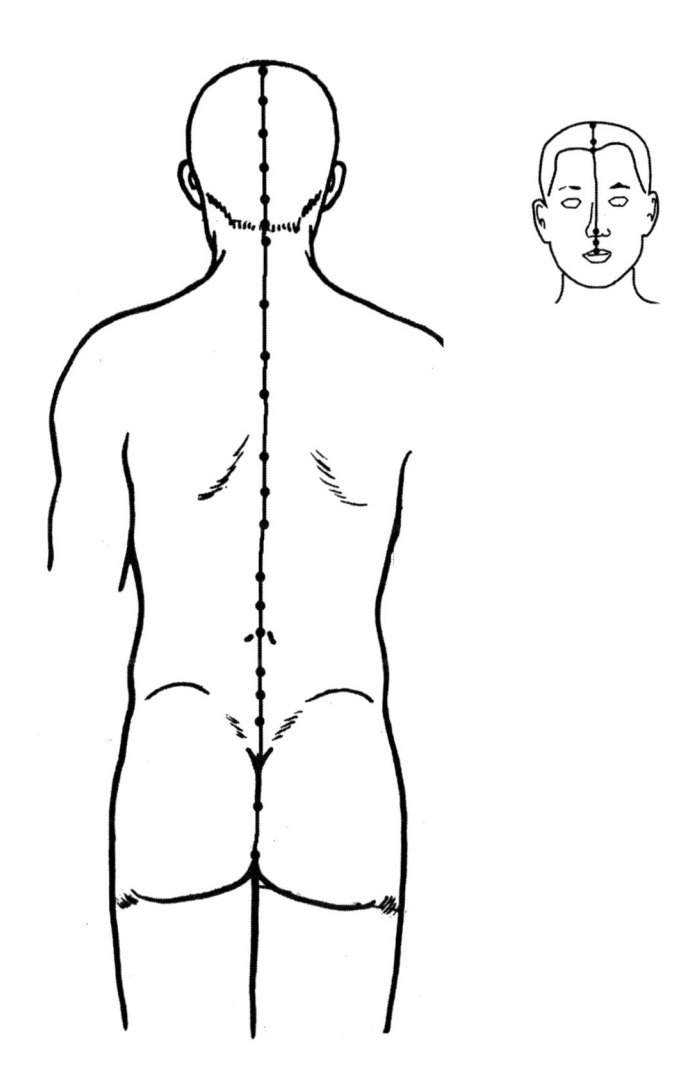

Du Mai (Governing Vessel)

REN MAI (Conception Vessel)

Ren Mai is considered to be the "sea of all the yin vessels" in the body. Ren 任, means to "take charge of", or "to accept" or "to take control." Because one of the things the *Ren* vessel takes control of is the fetus, it is often referred to as the "Conception Vessel." In this sense "conception" does not just mean to give birth but also to nourish life. Ren Mai is less a vessel than an area where yin and blood collect.[68] Both Ren Mai and Du Mai emanate from the Gate of Vitality, the *Dan Tian* and *Mingmen*.

Ren Mai commands the yin of the body – it is the "Sea of Yin" - and ensures free circulation in the yin parts of the body. Ren Mai regulates all of the yin channels in the body. It is the "Sea of Yin Vessels." The master point of Ren Mai is *Lie Que* ("Broken Sequence") – LU 7. The Internal branch of the lung meridian connects with and also runs parallel to Ren Mai, traveling from the lungs and chest down to the large intestine.

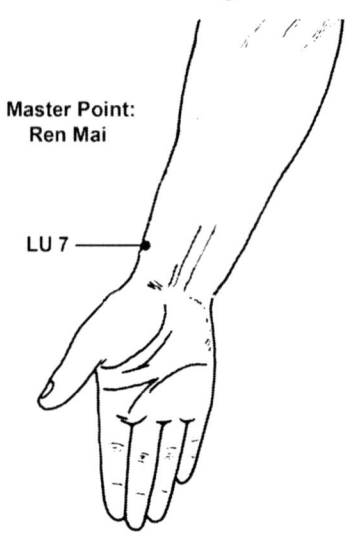

---

[68] *Applied Channel Theory in Chinese Medicine: Wang Ju-Yi's Lectures on Applied Channel Therapeutics* by Wang Ju-Yi and Jason D. Robertson. Seattle: Eastland Press, 2008, p. 289.

Ren Mai Functions, Connections & Associations

- Ren Mai emanates from the *Mingmen*, kidneys and genitals and emerges at the Huyin acu-point (Ren 1 in the perineum).
- In the medical texts Ren Mai is depicted ascending up the midline of the front of the body, ending at Ren 24, located between the lower lip and chin. In Nei gong texts it is depicted as descending down the front of the body.

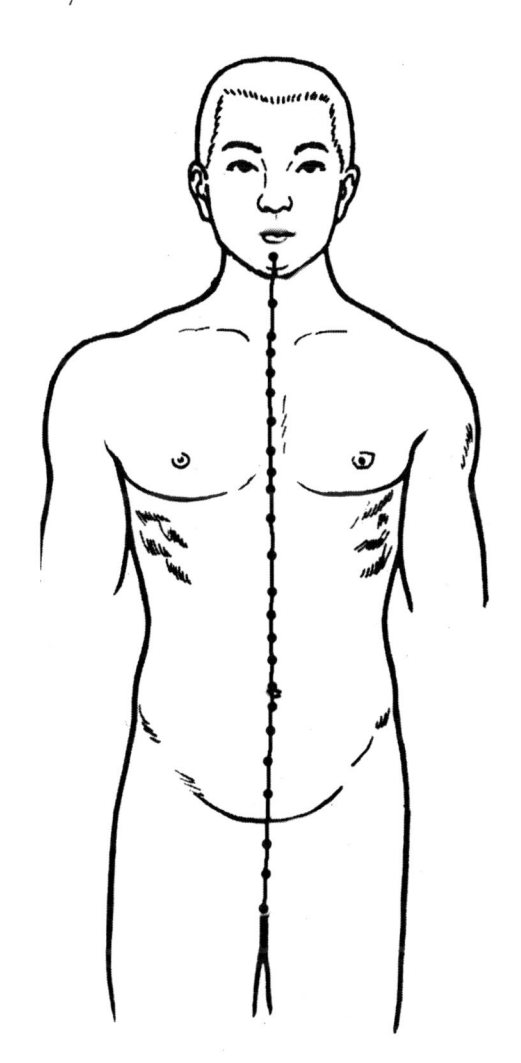

Ren Mai (Conception Vessel)

CHONG MAI (Thrusting Vessel)

Chong Mai is also known as the Penetrating Vessel, the Thoroughfare Vessel, the Vital Vessel.[69] Chong (冲) means "to rush vigorously," or to "surge". It can also mean "thoroughfare" or an open road - a pathway of communication. In this sense Chong Mai acts as a passage for free movement upward and downward in the body. The surging and penetrating aspects of Chong Mai emphasize its ability to connect and move.

Chong Mai is said to share a common source with Ren Mai and Du Mai - emanating from the *Mingmen* and the kidneys and descending to connect with both channels at *Hui Yin* ("Yin Meeting" Ren1). Chong Mai lies between Ren Mai and Du Mai. One branch of Chong Mai enters the spine at the sacrum and ascends at least as far as *Mingmen*. This branch is known as the "Sea of Channels and Vessels" and communicates with the rest of the channel system.[70] Another branch emerges at *Qi Chong* ("Qi Throughfare" or "Vigorous Street of Qi" - ST 30) and then follows the kidney channel upward to the chest.

Chong Mai connects *Qi Hai* ("Sea of Qi") in the Dan Tian with *Qi Hai* in the chest. Chong Mai connects with the pulsation of blood in the torso, integrating the flow of blood to the internal organs. It therefore links the Three Heaters (three parts of the torso). Through its branch that rises along the inside of the spine, Chong Mai connects with the *Mingmen* and establishes a link with the role of the Triple Heater in disseminating *Yuan Qi* ("primary" or "original" qi).

---

[69] *The Secondary Vessels of Acupuncture: A Detailed Account of their Energies, Meridians and Control Points* by Royston Low. New York: Thorsons Publishers Inc. 1983, pp. 154-55.

[70] *An Exposition of the Extraordinary Vessels: Acupuncture, Alchemy & Internal Medicine* by Charles Chace and Miki Shima. Seattle: Eastland Press, 2010, p. 234.

The "Sea of the Twelve Channels" is controlled by Chong Mai. This function is related to two braches of Chong Mai. One travels upward to connect with *Da Zui* ("Great Shuttle" – BL 11), the spine and brain. The other extends from ST 30, to the stomach channel on the lower leg and connects to *Shang Ju Xu* (Upper Great Hollow – ST 37) and *Xia Ju Xu* ("Lower Great Hollow" - ST 39).[71] Yet another branch travels from KID 11 down the medial thigh connecting to the bottom of the foot at KID 1.[72] It is likely through these latter two connections that Chong Mai reaches *Gong Sun* (SP 4), the "master point" of Chong Mai. These pathways connect Chong Mai to the energies of Earth through the feet and Heaven through the brain and vertex.

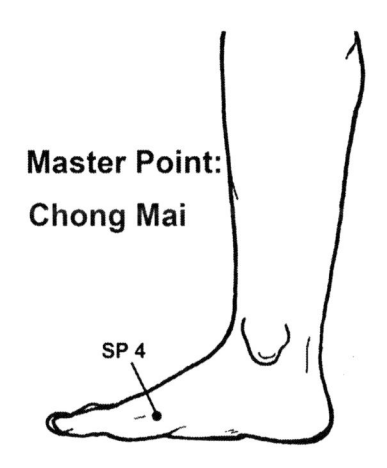

Master Point:
Chong Mai

SP 4

---

[71] *Huangdi Neijing Ling Shu: Books IV to V with commentary; Vol II.* Nguyen Van Nghi, Tran Viet Dzung, Christine Recours Nguyen. Sugar Grove, NC: Jung Tao Productions 1995 – English Edition 2006, p. 147.
[72] *The Acupuncturist's Clinical Handbook,* by Jeffrey H. Jacob, D.O.M., L.Ac New York: Integrative Wellness Inc. 2003; Sante Fe: Aesclipius Press 1996, pp. 244-46.

Chong Mai Functions, Connections & Associations

- Chong Mai is the "Sea of Blood."
- Chong Mai is the "Sea of the Twelve Channels."
- Chong Mai also shares the name "Sea of the Five Zang and Six Fu" (organs), with the stomach. This is because the stomach helps to replenish and renew qi and essence. Chong Mai and the Stomach have a strong relationship and work together.[73]
- The Liver and Chong Mai have a close association due to the liver's function of storing and releasing blood, and Chong Mai's role as the Sea of Blood. Both are involved in menstruation and the flow of blood to and from the organs of reproduction.
- Chong Mai connects to the face and chest and creates facial hair in men and lactation in woman.
- Chong and Ren overlap in their role of regulating blood to the uterus and reproductive organs. When a woman reaches puberty, menstruation begins when Ren Mai is passable (open) and the Chong Mai is full.[74]

---

[73] *The Eight Extraordinary Meridians,* by Claude Larre and Eisabeth Rochat de la Vallee. Monkey Press 1997, pp. 114-15.
[74] *Nan Ching: the Classic of Difficulties,* translated and annotated by Paul U. Unschuld. Berkely: University of California Press, 1986, p. 329.

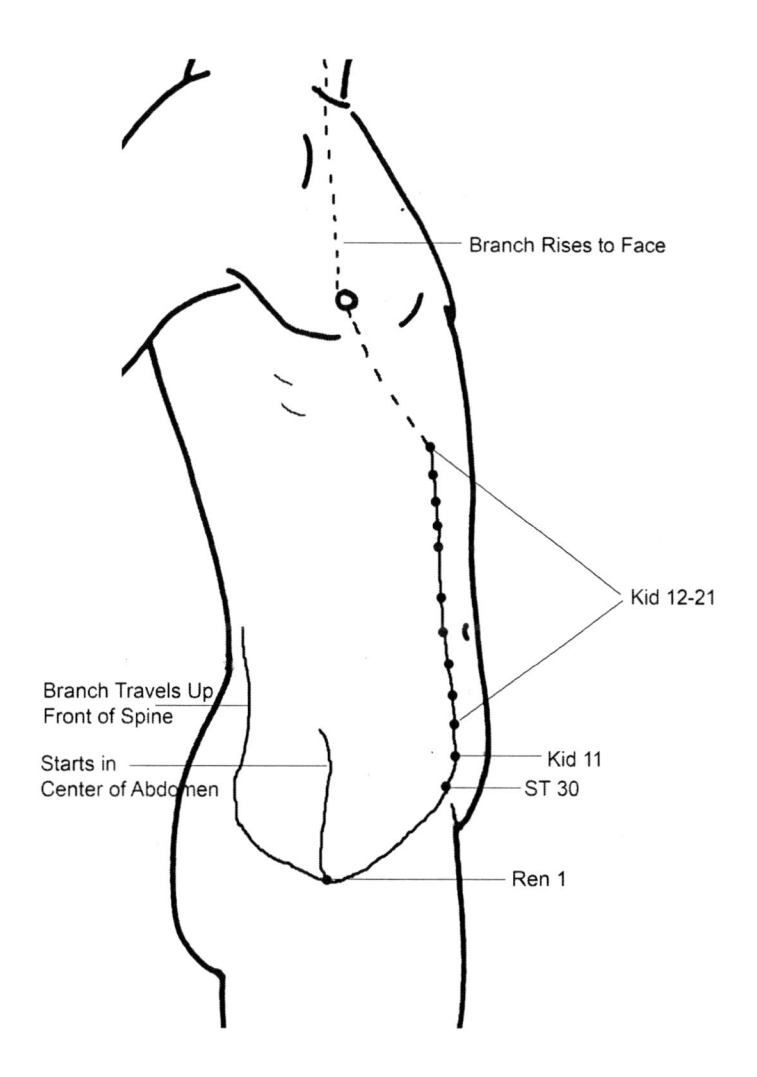

Chong Mai (Thrusting Vessel)

DAI MAI (Belt Vessel)

Dai Mai is called the belt or girdle vessel. Dai (带) can also mean a "strap" or "something that holds firmly."[75] Dai Mai is the only one of the meridians and Extraordinary Vessels vessel whose trajectory is horizontal or transverse rather than longitudinal. Dai Mai therefore connects the front and back of the body at the level of the yao and waist. Dai Mai also connects with all the other meridians as they pass through the waist, binding them together and connecting their energies. Therefore, it both regulates the other meridians and integrates upward and downward movement in the body. The classic symptom of a Dai Channel disorder is feeling as though one is seated in cool water with a feeling of cold in the abdomen. This may be accompanied by a feeling of weakness in the lower body.

Bao Mai and *Da Bao* are considered by some sources to be two sub-vessels of Dai Mai. The acu-point *Da Bao* (SP 21) "big wrapper" is also known as the "Great Luo Vessel of the Spleen." This collateral vessel emanating from the SP 21 acu-point, wraps around the chest to connect with the *Jiu Wei* "Turtledove Tail" Ren 15), the Luo of the Ren Channel. *Da Bao* also wraps around to the back to connect with the Du Vessel. This horizontal vessel is called the *Bao Mai* (wrapper vessel). Structurally, the *Bao Mai* forms a ring around the chest and thorax. It is analogous to Dai Mai and is sometimes considered an extension of Dai Mai. Classically Bao Mai was associated with both the acu-point *Da Bao* (SP 21) and *Yuan Ye* ("Armpit Abyss" - GB 22).[76] Some scholars like Nygun Van Ghyi feel that the Bao Mai emanates from SP 21 to form a ring around the outside of the

---

[75] *The Eight Extraordinary Meridians,* by Claude Larre and Eisabeth Rochat de la Vallee. Monkey Press 1997, p. 133.
[76] Channel Systems of Chinese Medicine: the Eight Extraordinary Vessels Lecture by Jeffery C. Yuen April 12 -13 2003. Copyright New England School of Acupuncture & Jeffrey C. Yuen. 2005. P. 143.

chest and thorax and that it emanates from GB 22 to form a ring around the inside of the chest and thorax. Others sources say that Bao Mai wraps around the frontal axis of the spine from the tail bone (at Du 1) to the "tail of the ribcage" (the xiphoid process at Ren 15).[77]

The master point of Dai Mai is *Zu Lin Qi* - GB 41 ("Foot Overlooking Tears"). This is the Wood point on the gallbladder channel which is intimately connected with Dai Mai.

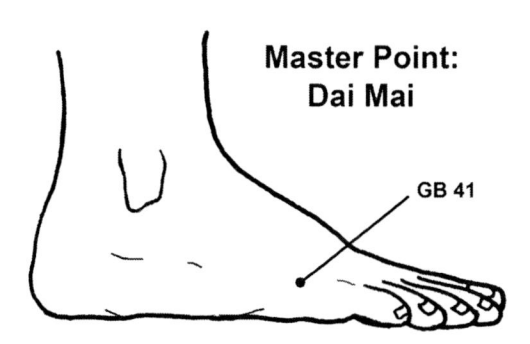

Master Point: Dai Mai
GB 41

Dai Mai Functions, Connections & Associations

- The Dai Channel has a close relationship with the Liver and Gallbladder meridians.
- The Dai Channel connects and helps regulate movement in the Ren, Du and Chong Channels.
- Dai Mai is the pivot between the upper and lower body.

---

[77] *The Acupuncturist's Clinical Handbook,* by Jeffrey H. Jacob, D.O.M., L.Ac New York: Integrative Wellness Inc. 2003; Sante Fe: Aesclipius Press 1996, pp.262-63.

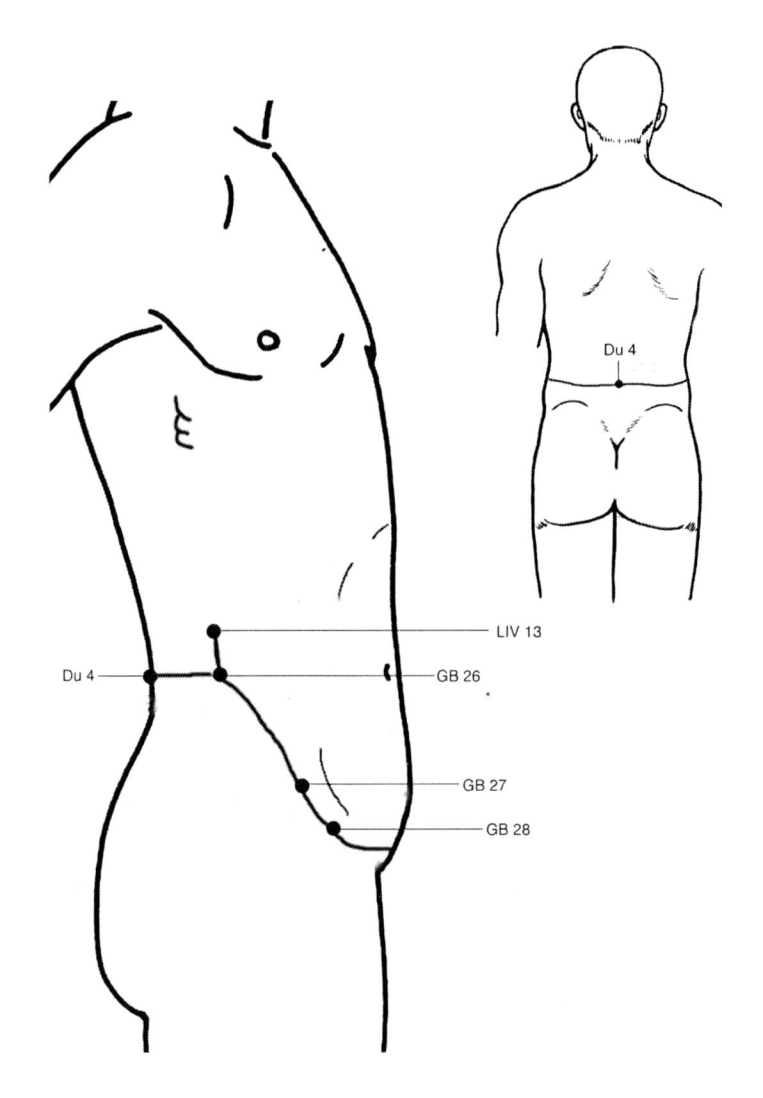

Dai Mai (Belt Vessel)

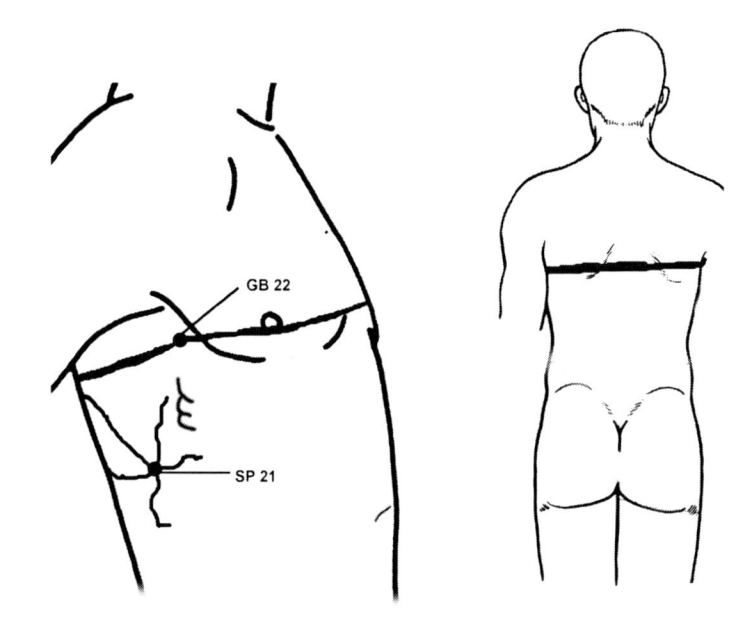

Bao Mai (Wrapper Vessel)

YIN QIAO MAI & YANG QIAO MAI (Yin & Yang Heel Vessels)

The character Qiao (跷) implies standing in a dynamic way with vigor and spring. Qiao can mean to lift one's leg or standing on tiptoe. This implies agility and movement, the ability to spring upward and lift up the legs in order to move. Both Yang Qiao Mo and Yin Qiao Mo start from the center of the heel and then split, one going up the inside of the heel and ankle and the other going up the outside of the heel and ankle. Ultimately the two channels rejoin at the corner of the eye – *Jing Ming* ("Brighten Eye" – BL 1). The Qiao Mai are concerned with movement and impetus - the movement of yin and yang energy ascending and descending from the foot to the head. Yang Qiao Mai accelerates yang energy into movement and Yin Qiao Mai accelerates yin energy into movement.[78]

Zhuang Zi tells us that the true man, the sage, breathes from his heels while most men breathe only in their throats.[79] This profoundly deep breathing of the sage comes from the movement of qi and breath up and down the Qiao channels. In Ba Gua Circle Walking Nei Gong, we walk and generate forward motion through the big tendon in the heel when using the mud-wading step while breathing deeply into the lower abdomen and even down into the legs themselves. This method of stepping both stimulates and balances the circulation and muscular tension in the two Qiao channels. Song Twenty-Four of the Thirty-Six Songs (mnemonics for correct practice of Ba Gua Zhang), references the importance of the heel vessels and their relationship to the Achilles tendon:

Power must be released fully from the bones and tendons,

Force comes from the bone and must be released by the tendons.

The big tendon of the heel connects with the brain and spine,

Promote power in techniques by using the follow step.[80]

Because the Qiao Mai are concerned with movement and impetus, they are linked with the network vessels (branches of the main channels and collaterals which enmesh the entire body), and transmit yin and yang between the interior and exterior. The network vessels regulate tension and slackness in the muscles and tendons. If one Qiao vessel is slack, then the other is tense. Usually this kind of imbalance occurs in the legs because of

---

[78] *Acupuncture Energetics: A Clinical Approach for Physicians,* by Joseph M. Helms, Berkely CA: Medical Acupuncture Publishers, 1995, pp.538-39.

[79] *Chuang Tzu: Basic Writings,* translated by Burton Watson New York: Columbia University Press, 1964, pp.72-3.
[80] *The Essentials of Ba Gua Zhang,* by Gao Ji Wu and Tom Bisio, New York: Trip Tych Enterprises LLC, 2007, p. 326.

the connection of the Qiao vessels with the ankle. However, this can also occur with the closing and opening of the eyes in sleep and awakening. This aspect of the Qiao Mai has a connection to the circadian rhythm. Chace and Shima observe that: *Yin Qiao nourishes the yin organs as it passes into the interior, while Yang Qiao nourishes the yang vessels and the striae in moving to the exterior.*[81]

The master points of the two Qiao channels BL 62 (*Shen Mai*: "Extending Vessel") and KID 6 (*Zhao Hai*: "Shining Sea") are located just below the internal and external malleolus. They are stimulated by the mud-wading step during Ba Gua Circle Walking Nei Gong.

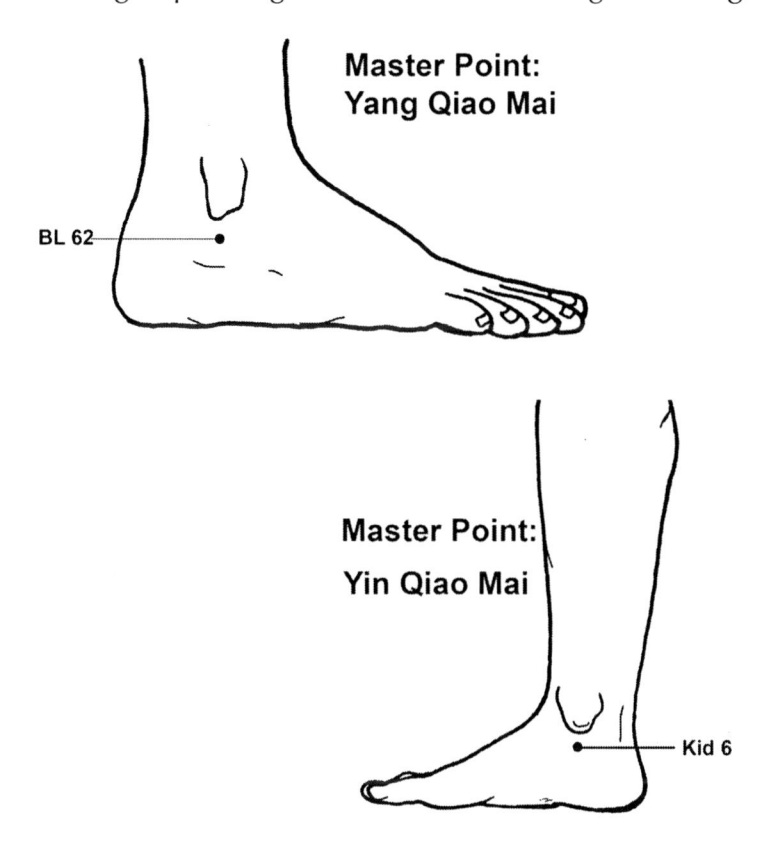

Master Point: Yang Qiao Mai

BL 62

Master Point: Yin Qiao Mai

Kid 6

---

[81] *An Exposition of the Extraordinary Vessels: Acupuncture, alchemy & Internal Medicine* by Charles Chace and Miki Shima. Seattle: Eastland Press, 2010, p. 220.

Qiao Mai Functions, Connections & Associations

- Because of its trajectory, Yang Qiao Mai has a connection with the Gallbladder Channel (Foot Shaoyang).
- Because of its trajectory, Yin Qiao Mai has a connection with the Kidney Meridian (Foot Shaoyin)
- The Qiao vessels help regulate the movement of the Wei qi in accordance with the circadian rhythm. Wei qi (defensive energy) moves to the interior during sleep - where it circulates among the internal organs. In the morning when one awakes it ascends to the eye and circulates in the vessels at the surface of the body.
- The qiao vessels govern and regulate the relative tension and slackness of the inner and outer legs
- The Qiao vessels aid upright standing and movement and agility.

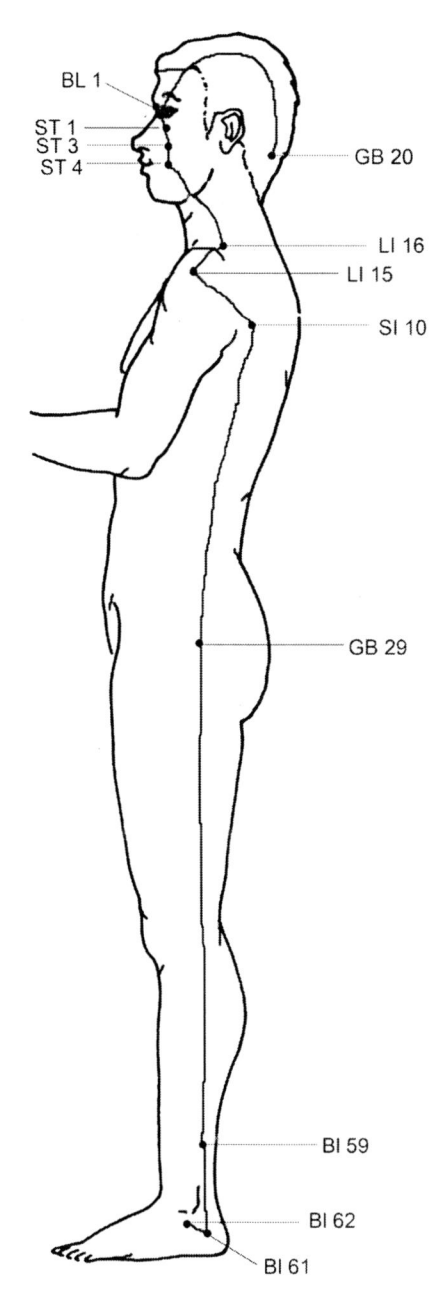

Yang Qiao Mai (Yang Heel Vessel)

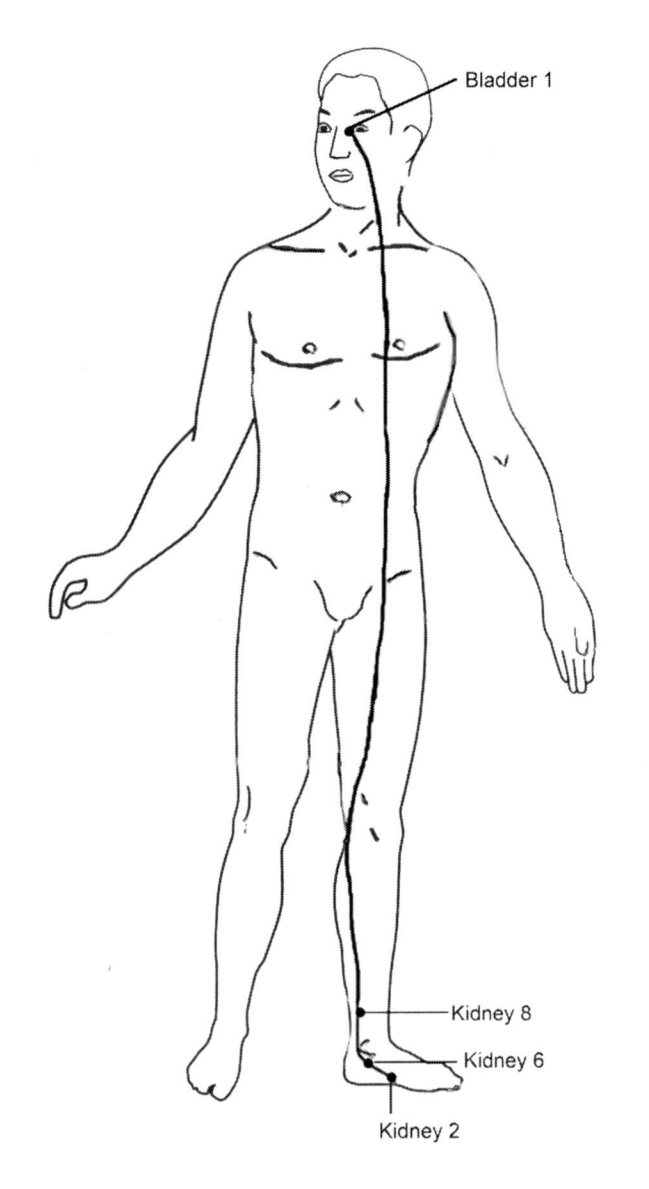

Yin Qiao Mai (Yin Heel Vessel)

YIN WEI MAI & YANG WEI MAI (Yin & Yang Linking Vessels)

Wei (维) means to tie up, integrate, or maintain. It can also mean to attach or link together, like a rope or a net. Whereas Qiao conveys the idea of rising up and putting into motion, the image conveyed by Wei is one of linking and supporting, like a great net or web. Yin Wei Mai links the yin and the interior while Yang Mei Mai links the yang and the exterior. *That which is moving circulating between all the yin meridians has the name of yin wei. And that which is moving between all the yang meridians is called the yang wei.*[82]

The Nan Ching (Classic of Difficult Issues) tells us that the *Yin Wei and Yang Wei are tied like a network to the body. The yang tie [vessel] originates from a point where all the yang [vessels] meet each other, and the yin tie [vessel] originates from a point where all the yin [vessels] intersect.*[83] The Nan Ching also tells us that the Wei vessels act like irrigation ditches and reservoirs that take overflow from the main meridians and circulate it to areas not nourished by the other channels and collaterals.[84] In this way they can irrigate, nourish and link the areas not nourished or connected by the other channels and collaterals.

Claude Larre and Elisabeth Rochat de la Vallee point out that in the quote above from the Nan Ching, no pathway is delineated for either of these vessels. They feel that the function of these two vessels – fastening and holding the body together and maintaining and balancing the relationship of yin and yang - is more important than the pathway.[85]

---

[82] *The Eight Extraordinary Meridians,* by Claude Larre and Eisabeth Rochat de la Vallee. Monkey Press 1997,
[83] *Nan Ching: the Classic of Difficulties,* translated and annotated by Paul U. Unschuld. Berkely: University of California Press, 1986, p. 327.
[84] Ibid, pp. 327-8.
[85] *The Eight Extraordinary Meridians,* by Claude Larre and Eisabeth Rochat de la Vallee. Monkey Press 1997, p. 215.

It is important to remember that in the Daoist conception of qi circulation in the macro-cosmic orbit, qi and breath circulate through the Eight Extraordinary Channels. Qi and breath move out from the shoulders along the outside of the arms via Yang Wei Mai and pass through the middle finger to the palm. From there, qi and breath return to the chest along the inside of the arms via Yin Wei Mai. Some sources attribute this flow to the *Yu Mai* (余脉) or "surplus vessels."[86] A branch of Yang Wei Mai, the Yang Yu Mai (yang surplus vessel), flows down the outside of the arm to connect with TH 5 and the middle finger. A branch of Yin Wei Mai, the Yin Yu Mai (yin surplus vessel), flows from the palm, through P 6 to connect with the chest. This Daoist Nei Gong description of the Wei Mai is not in agreement with the medical texts and is based upon an internal understanding of the channels.

The master point of Yang Wei Mai is *Wai Guan* ("Outer Pass" – TH 5) on the outside of the arm two body inches above the wrist. The master point for Yin Wei Mai is *Nei Guan* ("Inner Pass" P 6), on the inside of the arm directly opposite *Wai Guan*. When performing the Millstone Pushing Palm in Ba Gua Circle Walking Nei Gong, these points are stimulated by the positions of the arms. Additionally the wrapping, twisting action of the body sends spirals through the legs, torso and arms connecting and linking everything together to create a unified whole body power. This posture therefore links, connects and unifies the entire body by stimulating the Wei Mai.

---

[86] *Taoist Yoga: Alchemy & Immortality* by Lu K'uan Yu (Charles Luk). Maine: Samuel Weiser, Inc. 1973. and *Chinese Medical Qigong Therapy: A Comprehensive Clinical Text,* by Dr. Jerry Alan Johnson PhD. D.TCM, DMQ (China). Pacific Grove, CA: The International Institute of Medical Qigong, 2000.

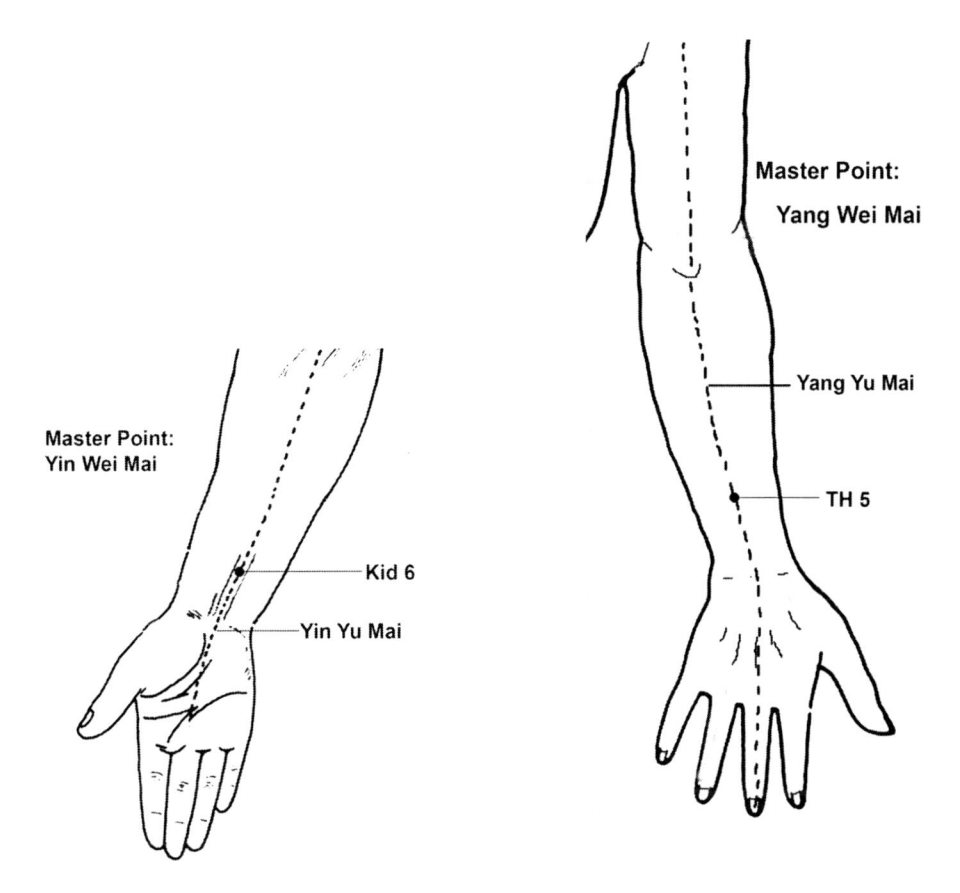

Wei Mai Functions, Connections & Associations

- Ren Mai and the three yin axes are linked by Yin Wei Mai.
- Du Mai and the three yang axes are linked by Yang Wei Mai.
- Yang Wei Mai connects with the Triple Burner (Shaoyang) and the yuan qi.
- Yin Wei Mai connects with the blood through Jueyin.

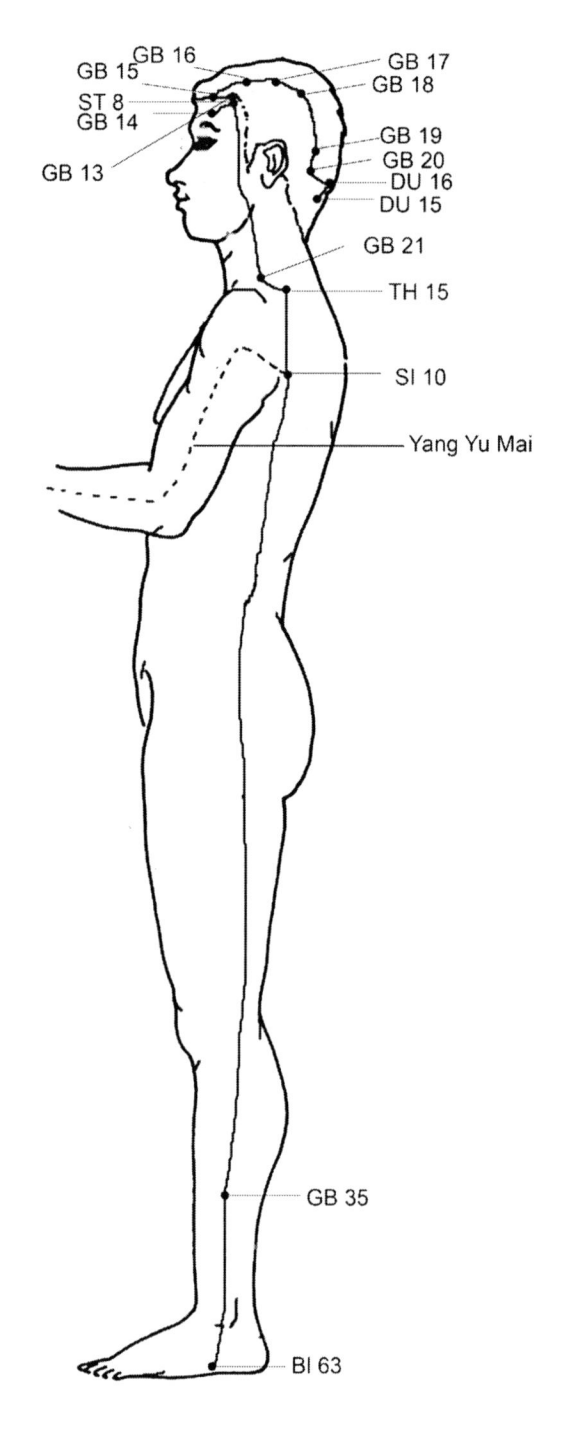

Yang Wei Mai (Yang Linking Vessel)

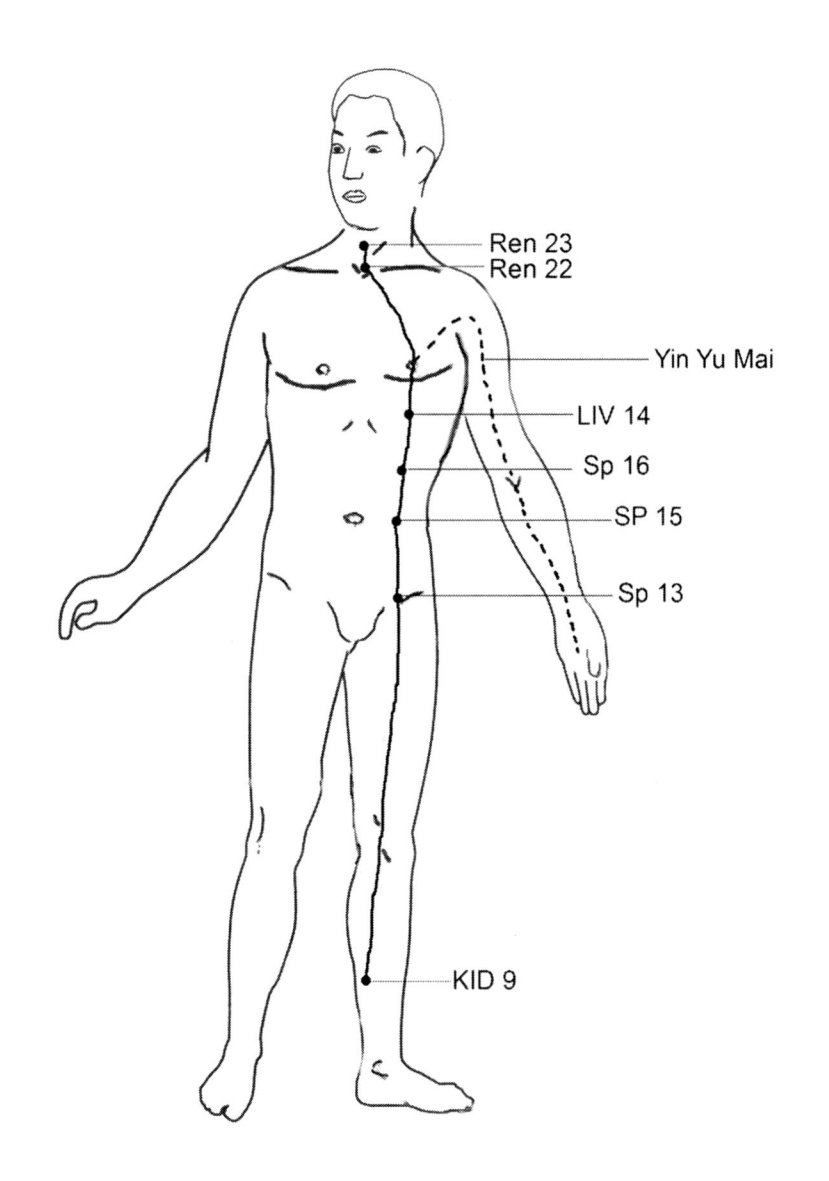

Yin Wei Mai (Yin Linking Vessel)

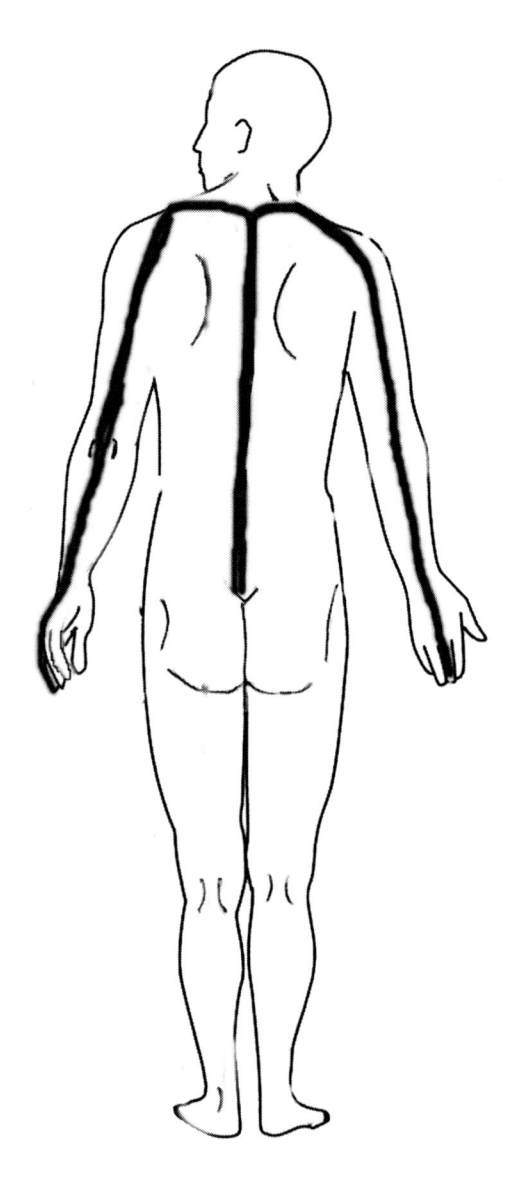

Alternative Daoist View of Yang Wei Mai

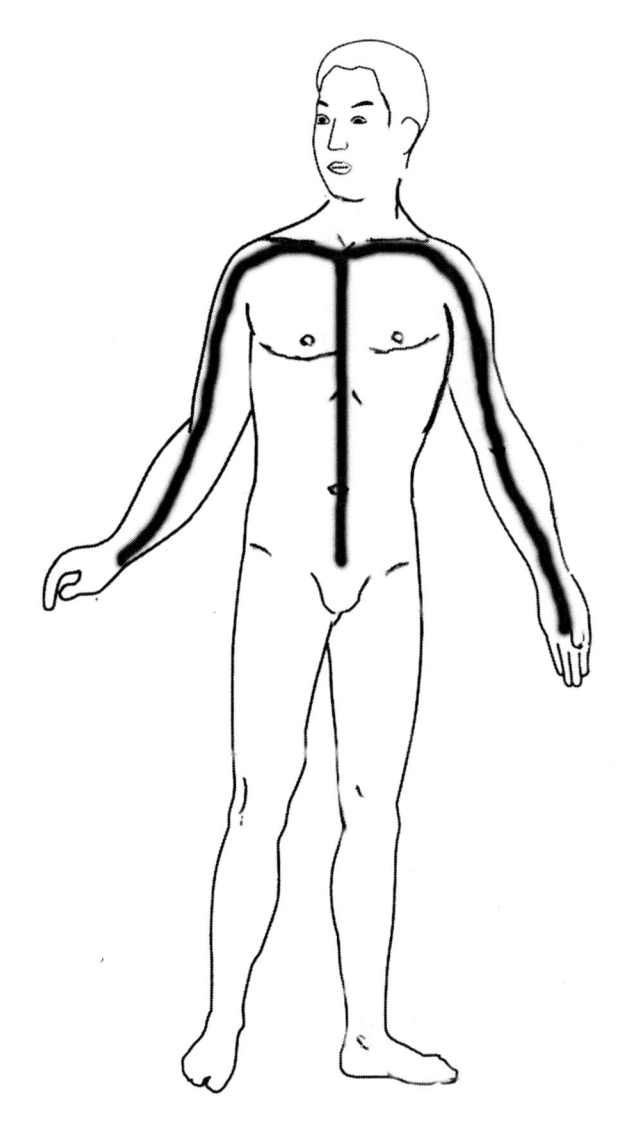

Alternative Daoist View Of Yin Wei Mai

The Eight Psychic Channels

The Eight Extraordinary Channels are also sometimes referred to as the "Eight Psychic Channels." This is due to their connection with the pre-heaven realm of human existence – conception and fetal development. Therefore they are thought to form a deeper, more primal matrix from which the other channels and collaterals develop. This matrix is also thought to engage on a deep level with psycho-spiritual aspects of an individual's life. In the West this has led some Chinese medical practitioners to try and make associations between the Eight Extra Channels and modern psychoanalytic theory. This is not how these channels are spoken about in China and it is the author's opinion that this obfuscates and confuses rather than enlightens. However, based upon their functions according to yin-yang theory, Chinese medicine, and Daoist inner-alchemical practices, we can speculate as to how these meridians may relate to human psycho-spiritual activity.

Du Mai

Du Mai, commands and regulates the yang of the body. Yang is related to movement, our intrinsic movement through life. Yang gives vertical strength to the body. As children we learn to stand upright, walk and move. This upright movement through life is a largely a function of the Du channel. Jeffrey Yuen says that *Mingmen is what throws and lifts the head up, and gets you into an upright posture. If the moving qi of the kidneys is held back, yang movement is hampered, preventing movement and stimulation.*[87]

---

[87] *Channel Systems of Chinese Medicine: the Eight Extraordinary Vessels* Lecture by Jeffery C. Yuen April 12 -13 2003. Copyright New England School of Acupuncture & Jeffrey C. Yuen. 2005, pp. 87-88.

The Du channel's association with the spine allows this upright and forward movement. Zhuang Zi (Chuang Tzu), in talking about nourishing life, tells us to take the Du as the regulating principle in order to preserve the body, nourish vitality and complete one's destiny. *The spontaneous fluctuations of behavior tend to normalize around the central current.*[88] The Du is hidden and unseen. Unlike the Ren, which lies in front, the Du is behind us and thus invisible.[89] *Hence it is opposed to the "knowing mind" and is the real controller, as opposed to the knowing mind's pretensions to control and direct life.*[90] Daoist Priest Kristopher Schipper, adds that *concentrating and regulating our own energies (qi) enables us to stand upright in ourselves, instead of having to lean against trees or on the crutches of systems and religious doctrines concocted by men.*[91] Only by remaining independent, by following the natural action of the spinal column, can we be a free human being, standing upright within our own vital space.[92]

Ren Mai

Ren Mai is the "Sea of Yin." It commands the yin of the body. Yang stimulates movement and yin nourishes form. Although Ren Mai is called the "Conception Vessel" because it connects to the uterus and interacts with conception and gestation, this is too narrow a definition. Ren Mai refers not only to the conception of new life, but to the nourishment of this new life and the nourishment of one's own life, with the same regulation and

---

[88] http://hackettpublishing.com/zhuangzi3.3 Additional Comments to Passage 3:3 in the Zhuangzi, by Brook Ziporyn
[89] Ibid.
[90] *Zhuanzi: The Essential Writings with Selections from Traditional Commentaries,* translated by Brook Ziporyn. Indianapolis IN: Hackett Publishing Co., 2009, p. 22.
[91] *The Taoist Body* by Kristofer Schipper - Berkely, Los Angeles: University of California Press 1993, p. 211.
[92] Ibid, pp. 210-12

protection as an embryo.[93] This is not only nourishing oneself but connecting with others, embracing, nurturing and being nurtured – the ability to establish relationships.[94]

Chong Mai

Chong Mai, the "Thoroughfare Vessel" or "Thrusting Vessel", through its connection with the heart and kidney, moves and disseminates the essence (*Jing*) and connects it with the *Shen* (spirit). This is the connection and movement of the source, one's nature, one's being and its expression in life. It is the jing, acting through the kidney qi, seeking fulfillment through the spirit. In this sense Chong Mai is the unfolding of one's constitution and archetypal nature.[95] Chong is *a great power, full of the seed and the promise of life animated with the vigor of the movement proper to life and the living being.*[96]

The great physician Li Shi Zhen emphasized the connection of Chong Mi with the spleen. The term *tai chong* may have originally referred to an emptiness or a void, implying a profoundly quiet and harmonious mental state.[97] This is the state associated with meditation. The descending trajectory of the Chong channel is thought to terminate at the instep, thereby connecting to earth, the center. This association of the Chong axis being grounded in the earth element, connotes a connection of the heavenly qi

---

[93] *The Eight Extraordinary Meridians,* by Claude Larre and Eisabeth Rochat de la Vallee. Monkey Press 1997, p. 87.
[94] *Channel Systems of Chinese Medicine: the Eight Extraordinary Vessels* Lecture by Jeffery C. Yuen, pp. 66-70.
[95] *Channel Systems of Chinese Medicine: the Eight Extraordinary Vessels* Lecture by Jeffery C. Yuen, pp. 46-7.
[96] *The Eight Extraordinary Meridians,* by Claude Larre and Eisabeth Rochat de la Vallee. Monkey Press 1997, p. 109.
[97] *An Exposition of the Extraordinary Vessels: Acupuncture, Alchemy & Internal Medicine* by Charles Chace and Miki Shima. Seattle: Eastland Press, 2010, p. 236.

with the earthly qi through the Chong, existing as an open and unblocked thoroughfare that is empty, harmonious and spacious.[98]

Dai Mai

Dai Mai and Bao Mai both wrap around and support the body. Dai Mai in particular also serves to interconnect the other vessels on the horizontal plane. The Dai vessel *is like a person's girding belt that in hangs in front and also closes and locks the essence qi. This is located in the spine and the entirety of the person's strength issues from here! That the spine is strong and not debilitated is nearly due to this lock.*[99] Both Dai Mai and Bao Mai act to secure and hold, like straps going around the body. They act as containers or wrappers that hold one's sentiments and deeply held ideas. Jeffrey Yuen believes they absorb excess, the excess and attachments of life.[100] Another way to view this is proposed by Claude Larre and Elisabeth Rochat de La Valee: *It is central and fundamental to the power of guidance and of holding something firmly and conducting well.*[101]

Qiao Mai

The Qiao Mai balance the tension of yin and yang on the sides of the body, particularly in the legs, our engines of movement. In this sense, they regulate and balance the polarity of yin and yang in the body and in life. The Qiao Mai are connected to our balance, our ability to stand and spring upward and outward. They have to do with our agility of movement. Like

---

[98] *An Exposition of the Extraordinary Vessels: Acupuncture, Alchemy & Internal Medicine* by Charles Chace and Miki Shima. Seattle: Eastland Press, 2010, p. 237.
[99] Ibid, p. 321.
[100] *Channel Systems of Chinese Medicine: the Eight Extraordinary Vessels* Lecture by Jeffery C. Yuen, p. 139.
[101] *The Eight Extraordinary Meridians,* by Claude Larre and Eisabeth Rochat de la Vallee. Monkey Press 1997, p. 134.

standing on tiptoe, we must balance so as not to tip too much one way or the other.[102] Jeffrey Yuen calls the Qiao Vessels, the "vessels of one's stance," meaning that they connect to one's viewpoint or outlook, to one's disposition in life.[103]

Wei Mai

The Wei Mai tie together, link, support, integrate and maintain the yin and yang vessels of the body. Integrity can only be maintained if things are linked together. While the Qiao vessels balance the polarity of yin and yang, the Wei vessels preserve the harmonious unity of the body by linking yin and yang into an organic whole. If yin and yang cannot maintain balance, if they cannot accommodate and support one another then there is a breakdown between movement and form, between activity and nourishment. Yuen describes this as connecting, linking and maintaining - a balancing of the outward questing movement of yang and the inward nurturing, connectivity and reflection of yin.[104]

---

[102] Ibid, p. 161.
[103] *Channel Systems of Chinese Medicine: the Eight Extraordinary Vessels* Lecture by Jeffery C. Yuen, p. 117.

[104] *Channel Systems of Chinese Medicine: the Eight Extraordinary Vessels* Lecture by Jeffery C. Yuen, pp. 99-100.

Chapter 9
The Eight Ding Shi Palms: Opening the Meridians
The Eight Ding Shi Palms and The Meridians

Normal walking, done properly, exercises and strengthens the whole body. Although the motions of walking seem linear, they are really a series of spirals and arcs that combine to produce forward linear motion. As we walk, the ankle rotates inward and outward and the arches of the foot flex and extend to carry the weight of our body as it moves forward. The muscles of the foot grip the ground, creating forces that move upward through the leg. The lower leg and knee internally and externally rotate sending spiral forces into the hips and back. The hips rotate along the axis of the spine, simultaneously rocking from side to side in a figure-eight motion which is transmitted through the ribcage to the upper back, shoulders and arms.

By walking around a circle slowly, steadily and evenly with the Mud-Wading Step, we maximize the spiraling forces that move through the body while balancing the muscular tension in the front and back and inside and outside of the legs. When you lift the foot so that the sole remains parallel to the floor and step it forward as though pushing a brick along the ground, you stimulate the kidneys by emphasizing the movement of the step though the Yong Quan (Kid 1) point on the sole of the foot. Stepping in this way engages the psoas muscles evenly and correctly. This opens the lower back, activates Ming Men and connects the lower body actions to the back and torso. Ba Gua circle walking strengthens the lower back and stimulates the kidneys, whose postero-medial surface is in contact with the psoas muscle.

The psoas muscle acts as a "rail" along which the kidneys can slide down to the level of L3.[105]

Sinking the tail and raising the upper back and the vertex in conjunction with sitting the kua and the stepping creates a gentle traction on the entire spinal column. This opens Du 4 (Ming Men) and stimulates the Ren, Du and Dai channels, as well as Chong Mai. Turning toward the center of the circle while walking in a circle creates multiple spiral forces that emanate from the foot. These forces ultimately flow in both directions, as upward directed forces coming from the foot and the step create countermovements that go downward into the lower body and foot as one step unfolds into the next. These spiral forces activate the primary meridians of the legs as well as the Qiao Channels through which energy moves up and down the body. The turning of the torso also engages spiral forces that open and activate Dai Mai and the Bao Mai. This creates free movement between the upper and lower torso and between kidneys and the heart, helping qi to move easily through Chong Mai ("Thoroughfare Vessel"). As qi moves up the body, relaxing the shoulders, sinking the elbows and softening the chest allows vital energy to flow into and back out of the primary meridians of the arms, as well as through the collaterals (Yu Mai) of the Wei channels.

The Downward Sinking Palm is the first palm that you practice because the position of the arms and body particularly stimulates and opens Du Mai, Ren Mai and Chong Mai. When these channels are activated and opened, it is easier to open the other meridians and channels.

---

[105] *Visceral Manipulation* by John Pierre Barral and Philip Mercier. Seattle: Eastland Press: 1988, p. 193.

Kan and Li: Water and Fire

In Chapter Two we discussed the importance of water and fire in Daoist practices and Nei Gong. It is worth repeating some of that discussion here. Ren and Du balance and regulate the cosmic forces of yin and yang and their expressions on the earthly plane: water and fire. Fire is represented by the I-Ching (*Yi Jing*) trigram - Li. Water is represented by the trigram – Kan.

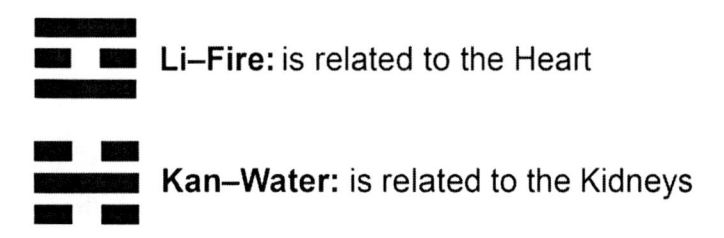

Li–Fire: is related to the Heart

Kan–Water: is related to the Kidneys

The trigrams are useful images in Nei Gong because they elucidate the relationship between the chest and the lower abdomen. Kan has a solid, yang line in the middle, so the lower abdomen (Dan Tian) is said to be "full" (of qi and breath) relative to the chest. Li has a broken line in the middle, so the chest is thought to be "empty" relative to the Dan Tian. These qualities attributed to Kan and Li are encapsulated in the following two statements which are used as a kind of mnemonic:

1. Solid (substantial; full) abdomen, unimpeded chest. (*Shi Fu Chang Xiong*)
2. Contain the chest (like something held in one's mouth) and draw up the back. (*Han Xiong Ba Bei*)

This is to some degree a function of "Kidney Breathing" that is essential to the practice of Nei Gong. Imaging the trigrams on the body in this way can be useful.

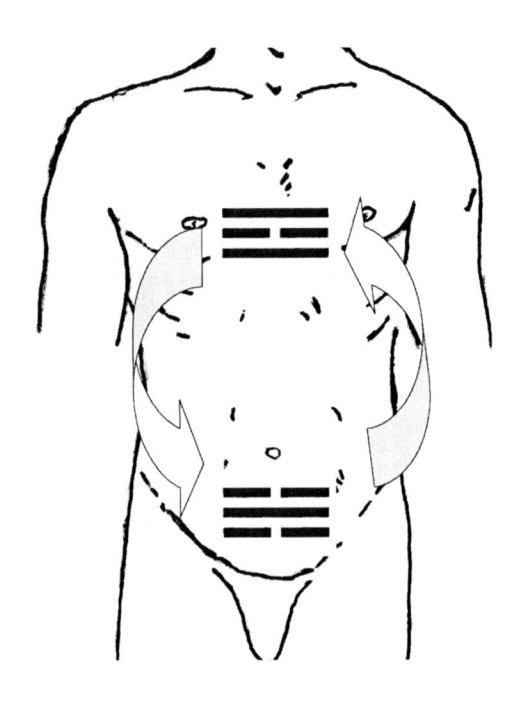

Water and Fire, Kan and Li, are not fixed. They naturally circulate and inter-transform in the body just as they do in the natural world. This movement involves the post-heaven energies of the five phases. Water in the earth nourishes plants and trees (wood). The sun's heat (fire) evaporates water so that it rises upward and transforms to become clouds – the highest point of yin. As yin coalesces, it forms water droplets and rain falls to fill the lakes, rivers and seas (water) and nourish the earth. This endless cycle also takes place in the human body. Qi, blood and fluids from the kidneys and spleen nourish the liver, and are transformed to rise up with the ascending and transforming power of the spleen and the circulatory power of the heart. Qi, blood and fluids moisten the lung, and are disseminated outward and downward through the tissues and organs by the cardio-pulmonary forces of the heart and lungs to return to the kidneys.

Water and Fire create a primal yin and yang balance in the body. Kidney water is like water in a pot. Under it is fire, the fire of the "moving qi between the kidneys," *Mingmen*. This fire evaporates the water which goes upward to coalesce in the upper body. From there it spreads out to moisten all the structures of the body, eventually descending again to the kidneys. The fire cannot be too hot, or the upward movement of heat and vapor will be too strong. If water is heated too much, it will dissipate and the body will be dry and scorched. If there is too much water, fire will not be strong enough to vaporize the water, or water will put out the fire. Therefore. this balance and the movement of fire and water must be harmonious

The balancing of Kan and Li that takes place when performing the Downward Sinking Palm is the first step in balancing yin and yang and the five elements within ourselves. To some degree, this is taking place in each of the eight postures, but the body-pattern created by the Downward Sinking Palm emphasizes the circulation of Kan and Li and the opening of the Ren, Du and Chong channels more than the other seven body-patterns of the Ding Shi. This is one reason why the the Downward Sinking Palm is considered to be the most important of the eight Ding Shi Palms.

Using the Eight Ding Shi to Open and Stimulate the Jing Luo

Each of the Ding Shi Postures opens a different Primary Meridian unit (yin or yang axis) and/or one of the Eight Extraordinary Vessels. By practicing the Ding Shi daily, while observing and attending to the specific meridians that the postures affect, the Jing Luo gradually open, unblock and flow freely. This in turn stimulates and strengthens the function of the channels, the organs and other structures to which the channels connect.

Generally, the order of performance of the Ding Shi is as presented in the following pages. The order can be varied, although one should always start with Downward Sinking Palm and end with Millstone Pushing Palm. Millstone Pushing Palm is practiced last because it activates the Wei Mai which irrigate, nourishe and link the areas not nourished or connected by the other channels and collaterals.

Body Unity

Although we can say that a specific posture, body pattern or movement opens, strengthens, or has an effect on a particular organ or meridian or more than one organ or meridian, it is important to keep in mind the unitary nature of Nei Gong and Qi Gon,. The basic alignments common to Nei Gong exercises and internal martial arts create effects that are felt in the entire body on many levels. The goal of internal exercises is to link the internal and external body so that even the smallest external movements create internal changes that travel and can be perceived through the entire body. Even when we appear to be just moving our arms, we are paying attention to what is happening throughout the body. So, while we can say that a specific body pattern like the Yin Yang Fish Palm "opens" the Dai Channel, we can also see how the position of the arms stretches the Small Intestine and Heart meridians while simultaneously engaging, opening and strengthening the Chong, Ren and Du channels. To give another example, the last three palms – Yin Yang Fish Palm; Heaven Pointing Ground Drawing Palm; Millstone Pushing Palm – all create a yin yang wrapping dynamic akin to a mobius-strip, but each with a slightly different orientation – one forward and backward, one upward and downward and one inward and outward.

Therefore, when we say that a particular movement or posture is associated with a certain meridian, organ or organ system, we are really saying that it has a tendency to do so, while at the same time it has other effects that can be felt throughout the body. In this book we will talk about how specific postures/body patterns have specific effects on organs and meridians as they are delineated in traditional Chinese medicine, but we must be careful of applying a mechanistic approach which may encourage us to focus too much on the specifics without keeping in mind the underlying unity. While one can "prescribe" or suggest alterations to the practice method based on individual constitutional and/or health concerns, ultimately we must recognize that in the context of the art of Ba Gua Zhang, the body patterns employed in Ba Gua Circle Walking Nei Gong are merely moments in time; positions that that one passes through as one changes and walks.

Important!

In the pages that follow, for each posture there is a section titled: "Pathways and Images." These sections talk about some of the ways that the specific posture works to open and unblock the Jing Luo it is related to. These images are meant to increase your understanding of the profound interconnections and logic of this Nei Gong method. They can be helpful, but any image should be attended to in a gentle, unfocused manner. Focusing too much on one aspect of the posture and its associated meridian(s) can cause the qi and breath to block, resulting in the opposite of what you are trying to achieve. If the images are not helpful, ignore them. Observing and attending to what <u>you</u> feel is more important.

Downward Sinking Palm

Downward Sinking Palm: Ren Mai & Du Mai

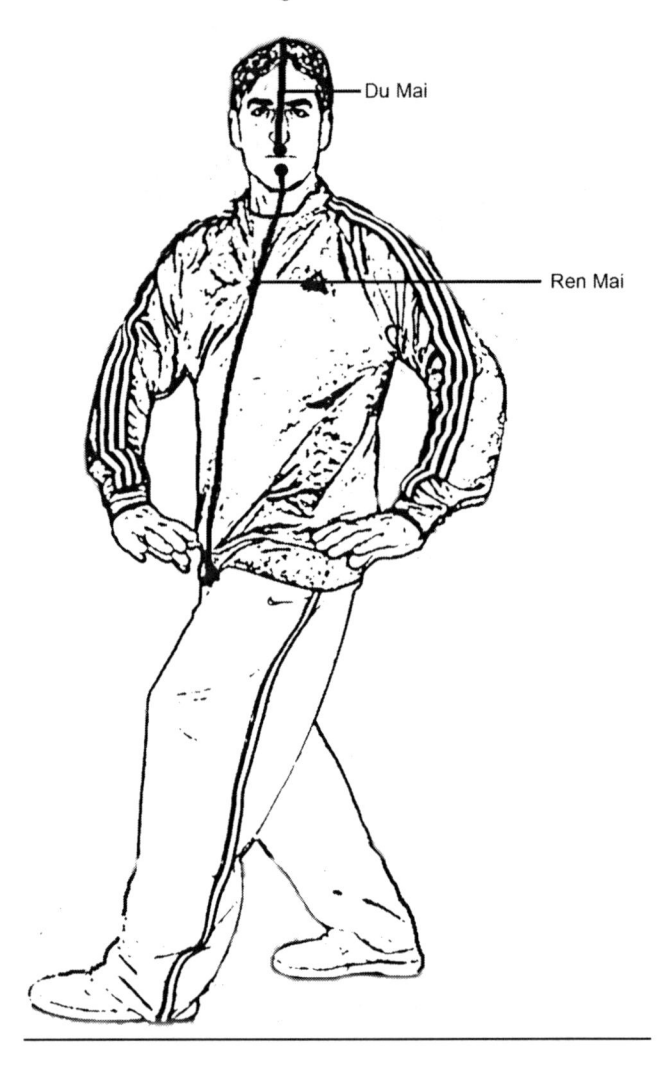

Downward Sinking Palm: Du Mai

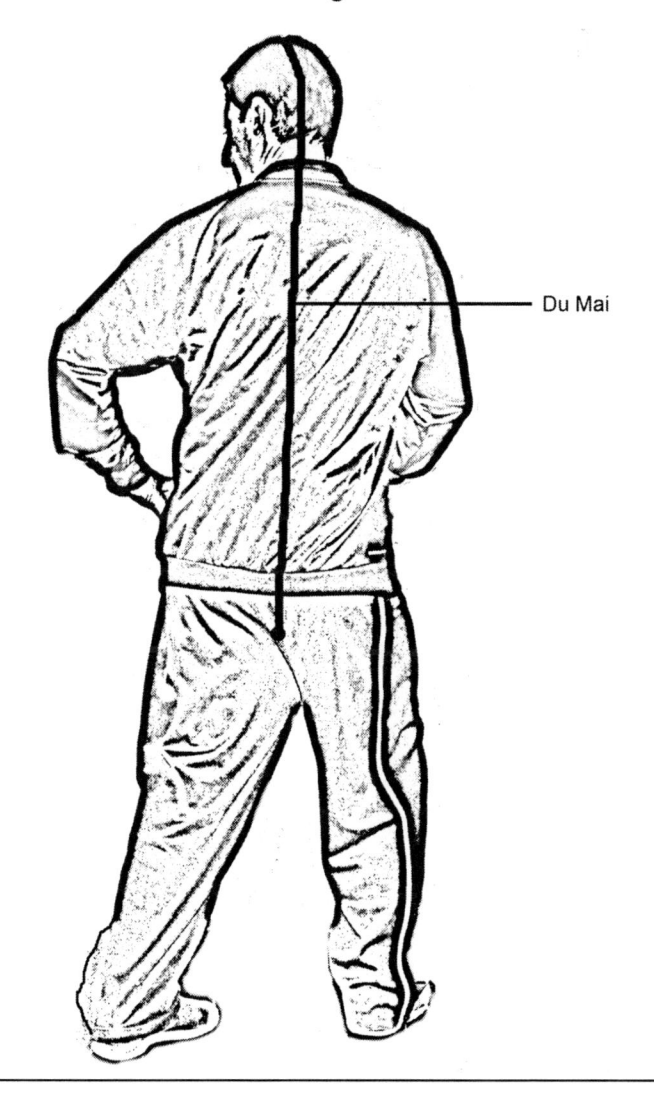

Du Mai

Downward Sinking Palm (*Xia Chen Zhang*)

Opens, Stimulates & Strengthens:

- **Ren Mai (Conception Vessel)**
- **Du Mai (Governing Vessel)**
- **Chong Mai (Thrusting Vessel)**

Activates the Micro-Cosmic Orbit

Circulates and Balances Kan-Water and Li-Fire

Supports and Excites the Triple Heater System

Nourishes the Dantian and the Yuan Qi

Pathways and Images

As you press downward to begin walking in the Downward Sinking Palm posture, it is like pressing down on one side of a rotating water wheel - as the paddles on one side go down, those on the other side rise up. As the wheel rotates, there is a constant rising and falling. In Daoist meditation, the image of the waterwheel is used to describe the circulation of Kan-Water and Li-Fire and the circular movement of qi and breath along the Ren and Du Channels – The Micro-Cosmic Orbit.

The round shape of the arms and the position of the hands also stimulates both SI 3 and LU 7, the master points of the Du and Ren Channels. The thumbs roughly point toward ST 30 (*Qi Chong* – "Street of Qi") where the more superficial channel of Chong Mai enters the Lower abdomen. An alternative name for this point is *Qi Jie* ("Qi Thoroughfare")[106]

---

[106] *Grasping the Wind: An Exploration into the Meaning of Chinese Acupuncture Point Names.* Andrew Ellis, Nigel Wiseman, Ken Boss. Brookline, MA: Paradigm Press, 1989, p. 84.

Moon Embracing Palm

Moon Embracing Palm: Hand & Foot Jueyin

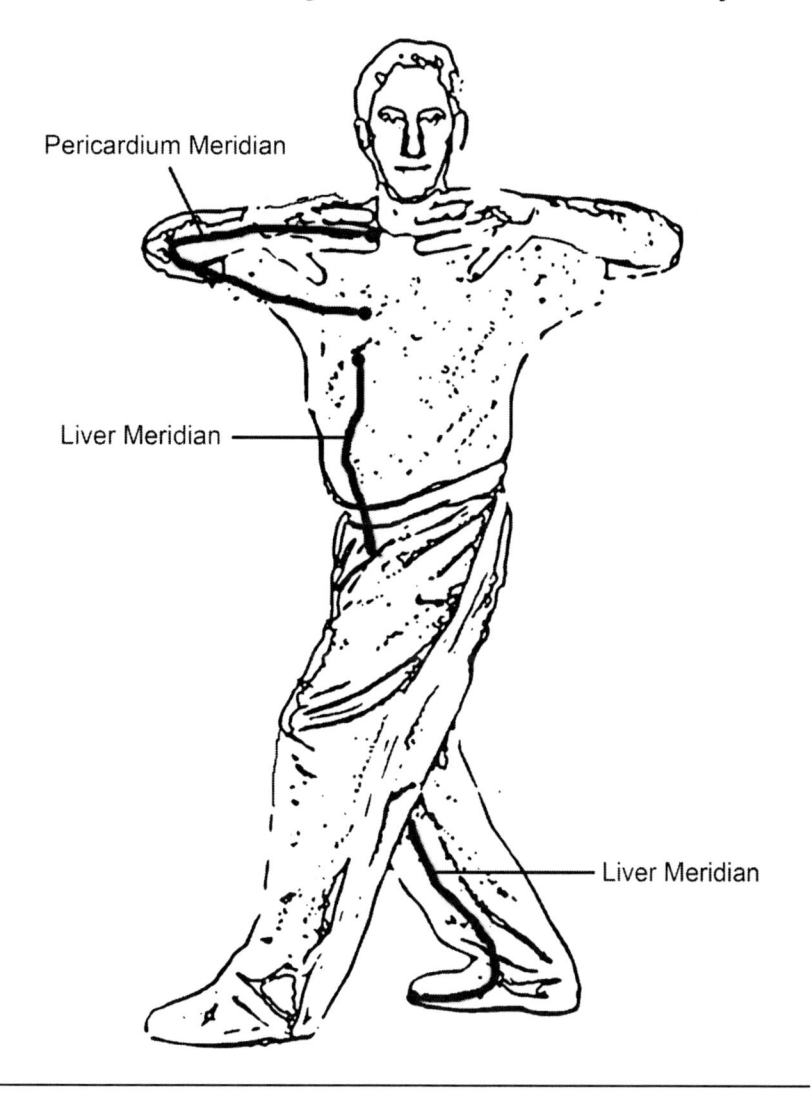

Pericardium Meridian

Liver Meridian

Liver Meridian

Moon Embracing Palm: Hand & Foot Taiyin

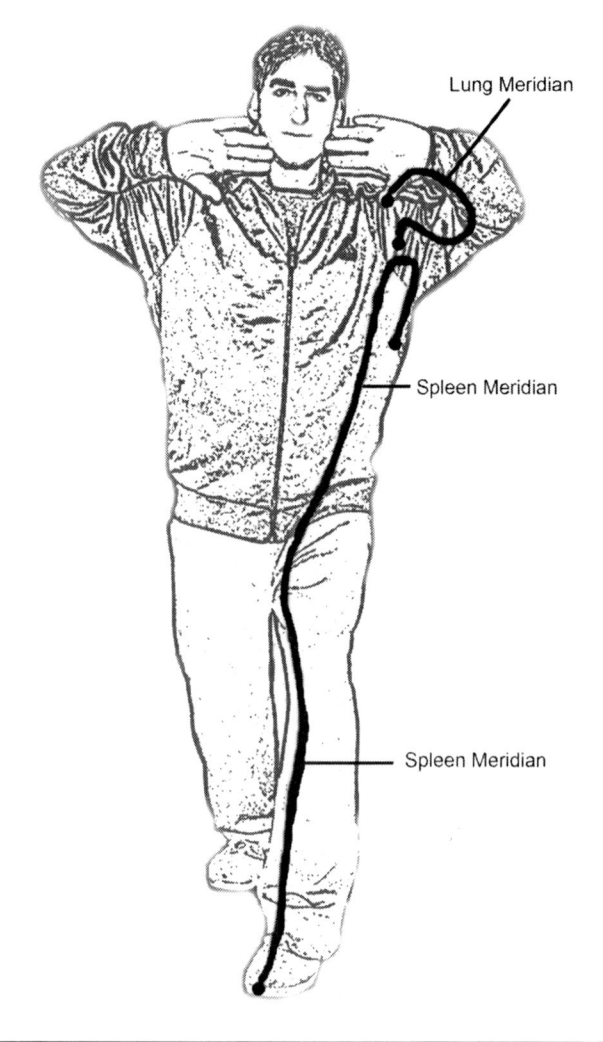

Lung Meridian

Spleen Meridian

Spleen Meridian

Moon Embracing Palm (*Bao Yue Zhang*)

Opens, Stimulates & Strengthens:

- **Hand and Foot Taiyin (Lung and Spleen Meridians)**
- **Hand and Foot Jueyin (Pericardium and Liver Meridians)**

Nourishes the Middle Burner

Pathways and Images

The rounded position of the arms opens the Lung and Pericardium Meridians. Qi and breath flow from the feet through the back and out along the arms, returning to the chest and back down to the feet. This current also simultaneously flows in the opposite direction. The position of the arms opens Ren 17, which connects directly to the Pericardium as well the area where the two Taiyin meridians meet (SP 20 and LU 1) and the area where the two Jueyin meridians meet (LIV 14 and P 1). It also opens SP 21. The spiral twist the posture creates in the torso also stimulates Liver 13: the *Mu* (alarm) point of the Spleen. The position of the arms, opens LI 4, a gate point for energy going to the fingertips, important points on the Pericardium Meridian (P 6 and P 8), and points on the Lung Meridian (like LU 3, 7, 8, 9, and 10).

Heaven Upholding Palm

Heaven Upholding Palm: Foot Yangming

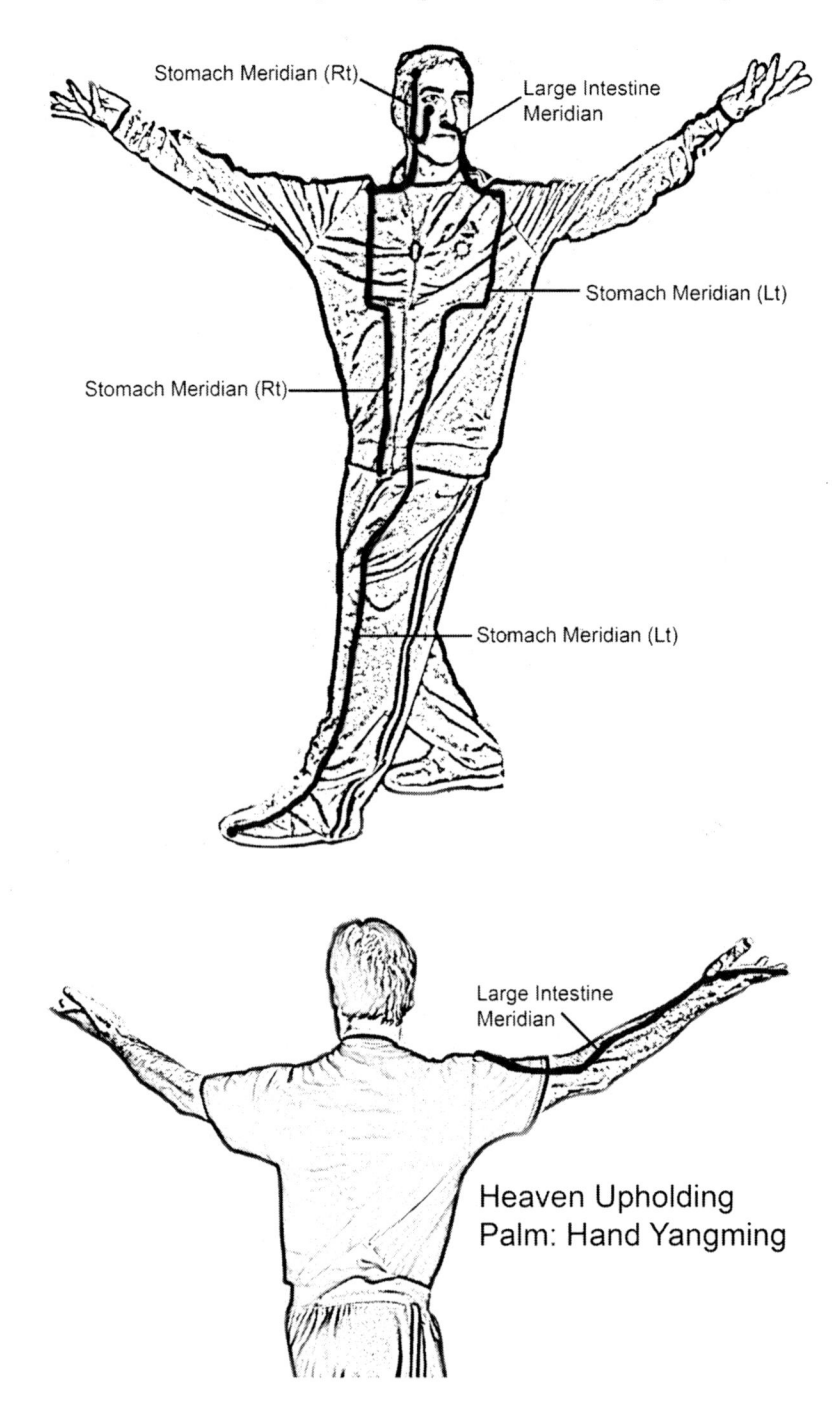

- Stomach Meridian (Rt)
- Large Intestine Meridian
- Stomach Meridian (Lt)
- Stomach Meridian (Rt)
- Stomach Meridian (Lt)

- Large Intestine Meridian

Heaven Upholding Palm: Hand Yangming

Heaven Upholding Palm (*Tuo Tian Zhang*)

Opens, Stimulates & Strengthens:
- **Hand Yangming (Large Intestine Meridian)**
- **Foot Yangming (Stomach Meridian)**

Benefits the Abdominal Organs

Replenishes Yin and Yang

Pathways and Images

The lifting of the arms in the Heaven Upholding Palm, in conjunction with the loosening of the shoulders, opens and relaxes the ST 12 acu-point, an important junction of several meridians including the Stomach and Large Intestine meridians and their internal branches. The position of the arms also opens the Large Intestine meridian's pathway in the arms, and the Stomach meridian where it runs through the chest and abdomen. The hollow palm and opening of the thumb and forefinger opens *He Gu* (LI 4).

Lifting the arms and simultaneously sinking the tailbone and relaxing the low back create a sensation of freeing the internal organs so that they relax. By practicing this posture daily, tension in the chest and diaphragm is gradually dispelled. Chest tension can create physical tension in the organs. The liver, gallbladder and stomach may feel as though they are lifted and suspended. Traditionally, this is sometimes referred to as "lifting the heart and hanging the gallbladder" and creates a feeling of "roasted lung and fried liver"[107] – ie: anxiety and worry and a sense of constriction or tension in the diaphragm stomach and chest.

---

[107] *Science of Internal Strength Boxing*, by Zhang Nai Qi (1933). Translated by Marcus Brinkman Taipei, Taiwan , 2005, pp.17-18.

Relaxing the chest naturally helps the circulation of water and fire and the sinking of qi to the Dantian. This also frees up the diaphragm - to which the liver, esophagus, stomach and intestines all attach - thereby aiding the downward peristaltic movement of the stomach and intestines and benefiting the internal organs.

Ball Rolling Palm

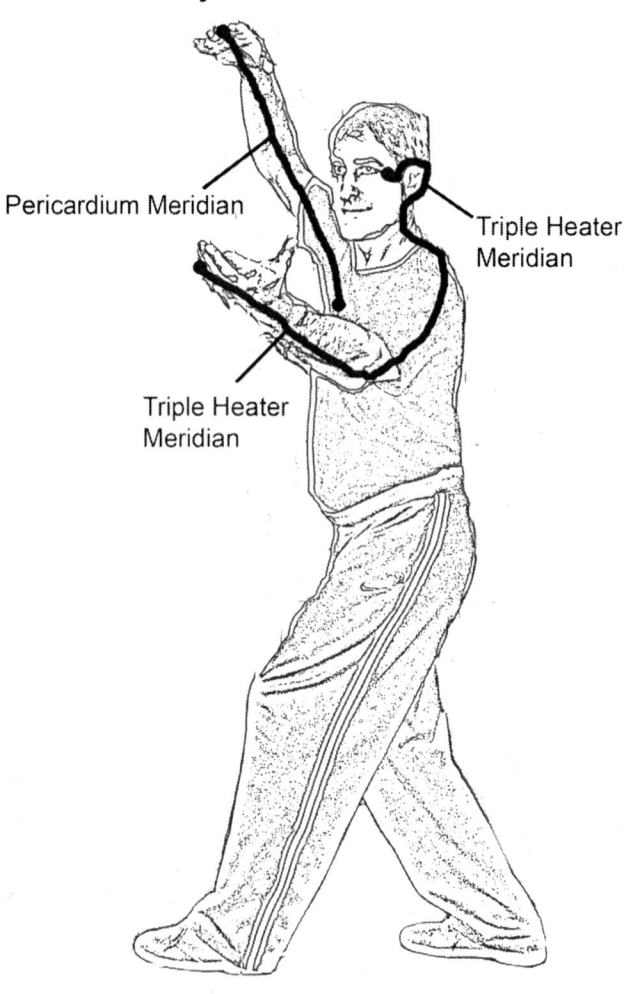

Ball Rolling Palm: Hand Shaoyang & Hand Jueyin

Pericardium Meridian

Triple Heater Meridian

Triple Heater Meridian

Ball Rolling Palm (*Gun Qiu Zhang*)

Opens, Stimulates & Strengthens:
- **Hand Jueyin (Pericardium Meridian)**
- **Hand Shaoyang (Triple Heater Meridian)**

Supports and Nourishes the Five Phases

Helps with Wind Disease

Pathways and Images

Through its rounded shape and image of holding and rolling a large ball, this posture creates a circuit through the arms, chest and upper back that connect the Pericardium and Triple Heater Meridians. This circuit runs in both directions, along the inside and the outside of the arms. The outer part of this circuit includes the upper back and the inner part the chest.

Although both meridians are associated with the fire element, Hand Jueyin is associated with the heart and chest while the internal branch of Hand Shaoyang ultimately emanates from the *Mingmen* ("life-gate fire," "the moving qi between the kidneys"). Therefore, although the rounded shape of the posture appears at first glance to involve only the upper body, one can also see and feel the ball-shaped curve that starts at the foot, goes through the buttocks, back and kidneys and connects to the arms.

P 1 is lifted and opened in the chest and points all along both the Pericardium and Triple Heater meridian are stimulated – P 4, P 5, P 7, P 8, P 9 and TH 2, TH 3, TH 5, TH 6, TH 9, TH 14, TH 15. Areas of the neck and nape through which wind can enter, and which also dispel internal wind, can also open and unblock so that wind can be expelled. For example: GB 20, DU 16, BL 10, TH 16, DU 14.

Spear Upholding Palm

Spear Upholding Posture: Hand & Foot Shaoyin

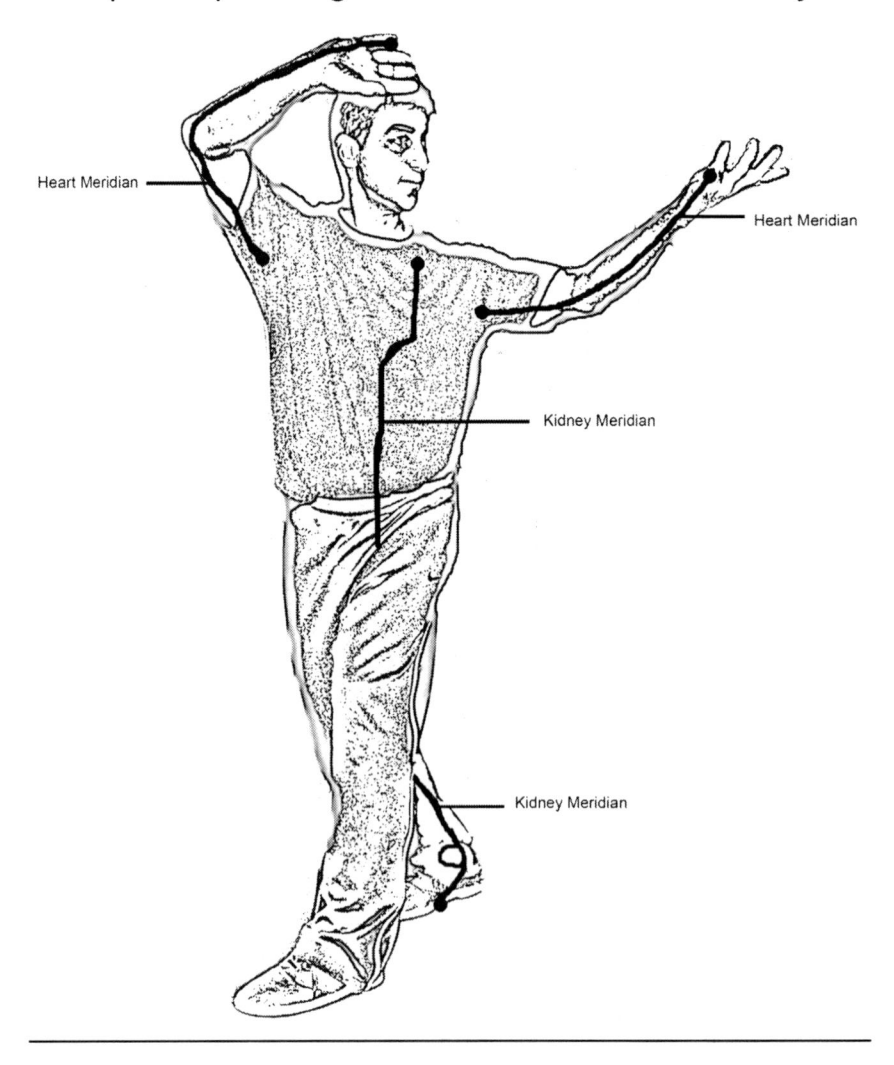

Spear Upholding Palm: Hand & Foot Taiyang

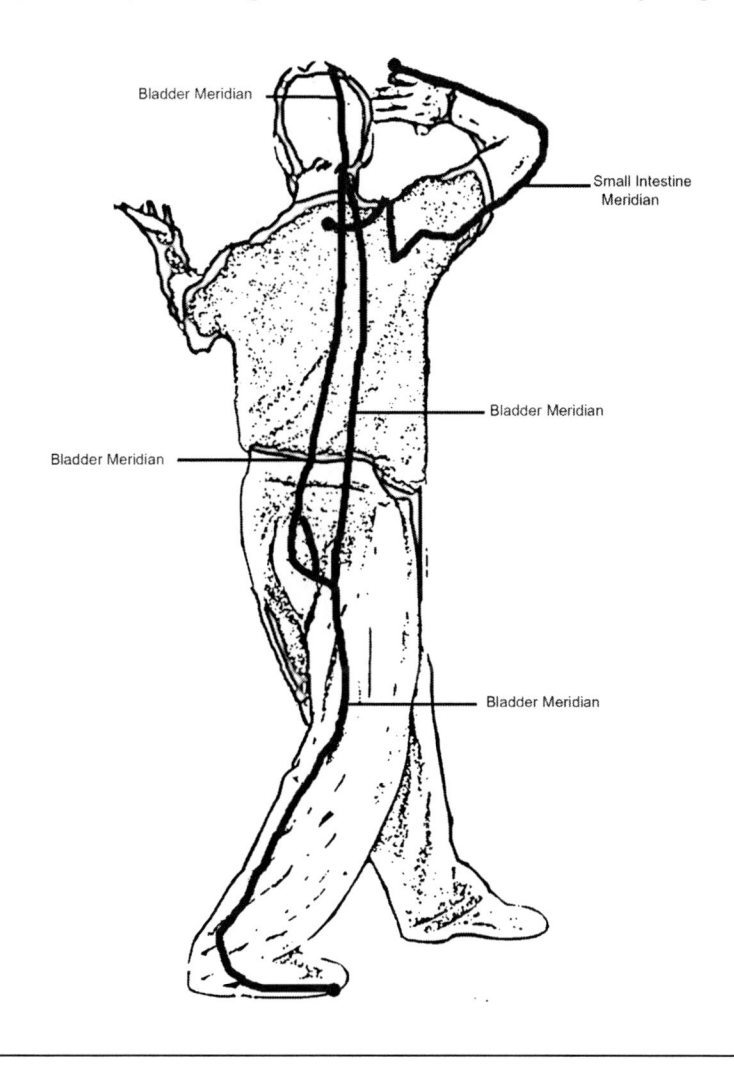

Spear Upholding Palm (*Qiang Tuo Zhang*)

Opens, Stimulates & Strengthens:

- **Hand and Foot Taiyang (Small Intestine and Bladder Meridians)**
- **Hand and Foot Shaoyin (Heart and Kidney Meridians)**

Supports the Triple Heater System

Pathways and Images

This posture creates a great spiral circuit which rises from the heel, goes up the Bladder Meridian on the back of the leg to Mingmen and the kidney area in the low back. From there it continues up to the shoulder blade and out into the arm and hand via the Small Intestine Meridian, returning to the chest along the Heart Meridian. It then travels to the foot along the front of the body and inside of the leg via the Kidney Meridian. This circuit simultaneously flows in both directions.

The arm that is raised overhead (the outside arm) opens and slightly stretches both the Heart and Small Intestine meridians. It also opens the cavity in which the heart rests, as well as opening the HT 1 acu-point. Further, this position opens SI 11 – a "gate point" on the shoulder blade which regulates the flow of yang energy into the arms. The part of the Kidney Meridian pathway that passes through the chest to connect with the heart is also opened up by the position of the raised arm. At the same time, the raised arm, combined with turning the body, creates a spiral pulling force that tugs on the kidney and *Mingmen*, as well as a number of the back Shu points. This spiral helps pull the right foot forward to hook (Kou Bu) as you walk around the circle, but the spiral also continues downward along the Bladder Meridian to the heel of the opposite foot.

The other (inside) arm balances and stabilizes the opening actions of the outside arm. It helps to create the spiral twist that runs through the body and also activates the Heart and Small Intestine Meridians.

Heaven Pointing Ground Drawing Palm

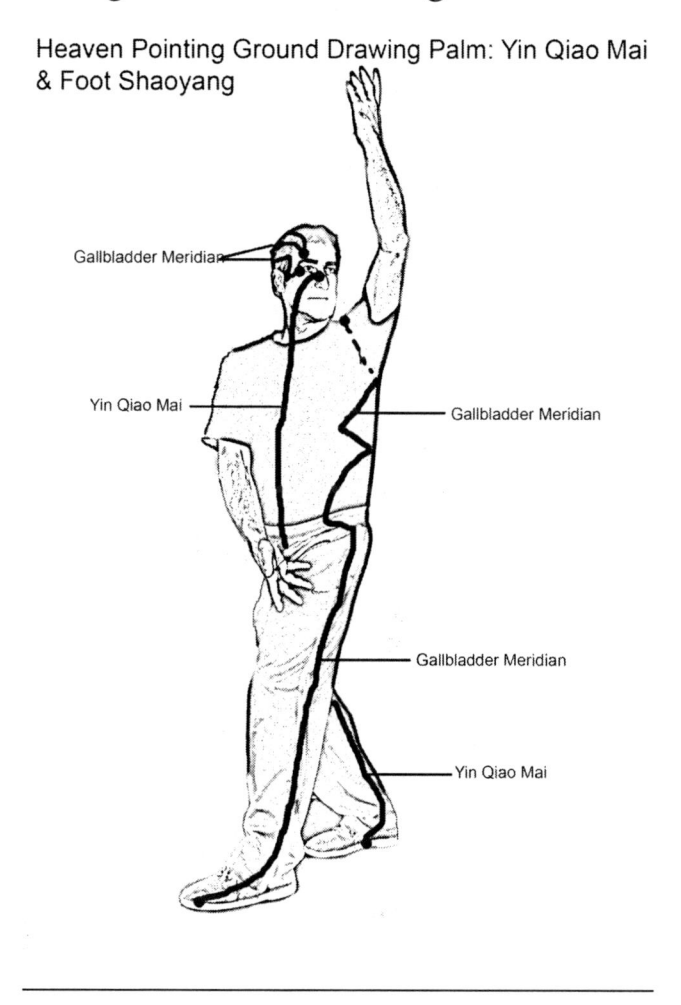

Heaven Pointing Ground Drawing Palm: Yin Qiao Mai & Foot Shaoyang

Gallbladder Meridian

Yin Qiao Mai

Gallbladder Meridian

Gallbladder Meridian

Yin Qiao Mai

Heaven Pointing Earth Drawing Palm: Yang Qiao Mai

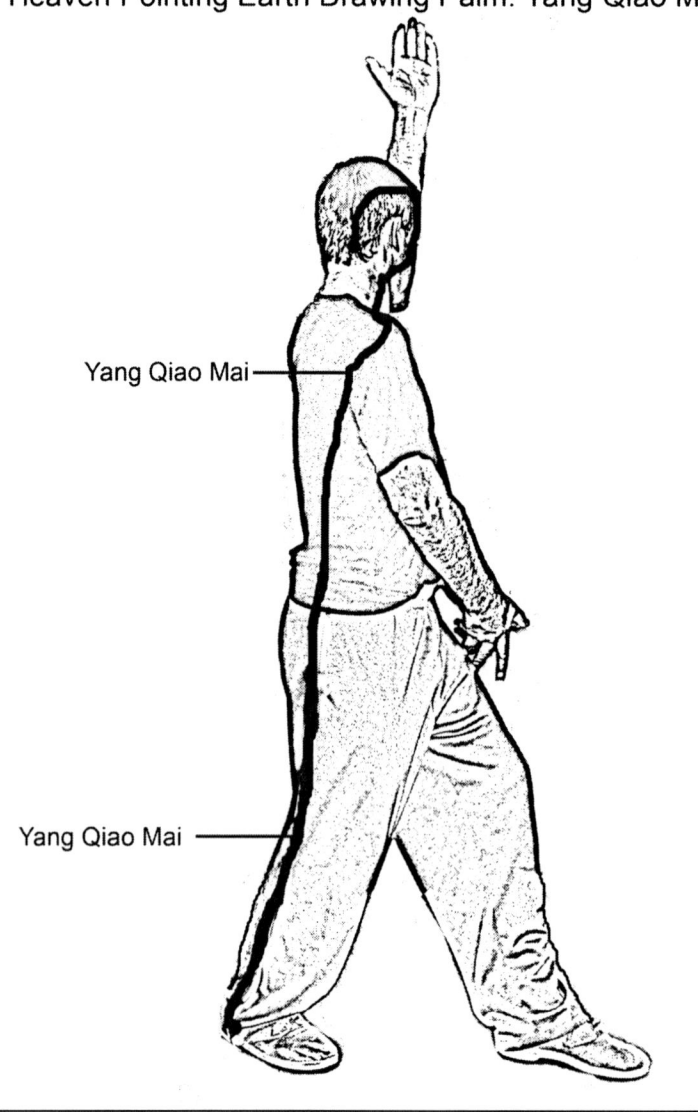

Yang Qiao Mai

Yang Qiao Mai

Heaven Pointing Earth Drawing Palm (*Zhi Tian Hua Di Zhang*)

Opens, Stimulates & Strengthens:
- **Yin Qiao Mai (Yin Heel Channel)**
- **Yang Qiao Mai (Yang Heel Channel)**
- **Foot Shaoyang (Gallbladder Meridian)**

Supports the "Hundred Meridians"

Strengthens the Spirit (*Shen*)

Pathways and Images

The yin yang balance created by the posture of Pointing at Heaven and Drawing on the Ground - one arm high, one low, one facing forward and one facing backward - puts a twist through the entire body, starting at the Achilles tendon at the heel and proceeding upward to the crown and heaven pointing arm. This creates a continuous looped figure-eight or mobius-strip connection between the two Qiao Channels. KID 6 and BL 62, the master points of the Qiao Channels, are a lifted and opened by the posture. The eyes are also stimulated by walking in this posture.

This posture opens the Gallbladder Meridian by stretching and opening the sides of the body. Even the portion of the Gallbladder Meridian's trajectory which passes under the scapula from GB 21 to GB 22 is opened by the raised and rotated position of the upper arm.

The connection between the spirit (*shen*) and the Qiao Mai is referred to by Zhang Bo Duan, a Taoist who wrote on Daoist internal alchemy in the 11th century. Zhang says that only when Yin Qiao becomes activated will the other vessels open. He refers to Yin Qiao as the "Governor of the Spirit" and the "Peach of Well-Being."[108]

Yin Yang Fish Palm

Yin Yang Fish Palm - Dai Mai & Bao Mai

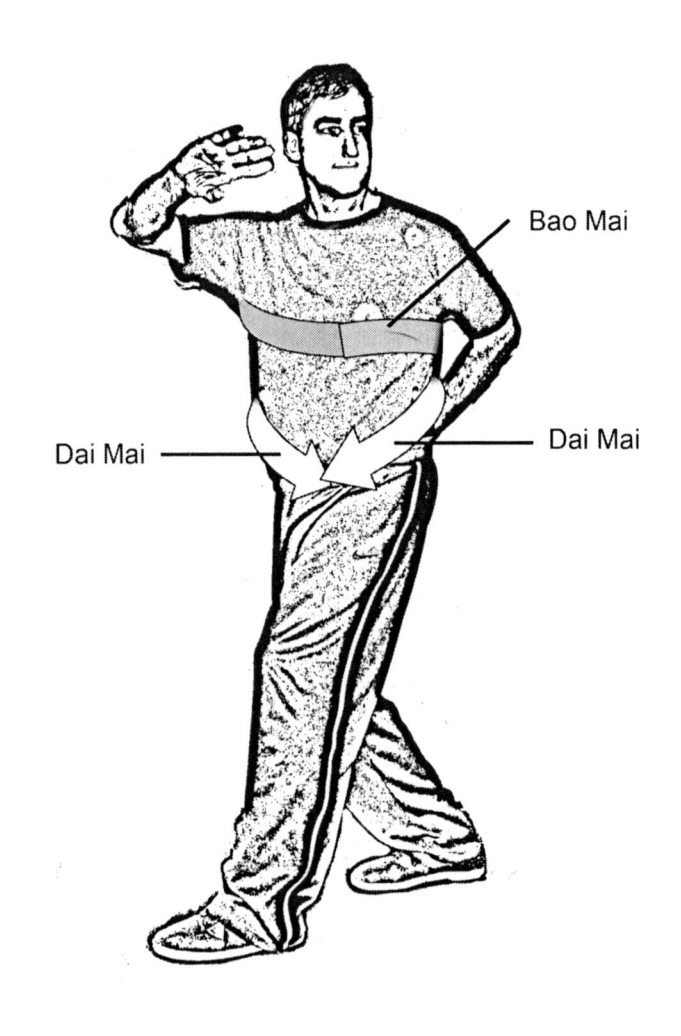

---

[108] *An Exposition of the Extraordinary Vessels: Acupuncture, Alchemy & Internal Medicine* by Charles Chace and Miki Shima. Seattle: Eastland Press, 2010, p. 110.

Yin Yang Fish Palm: Dai Mai & Bao Mai

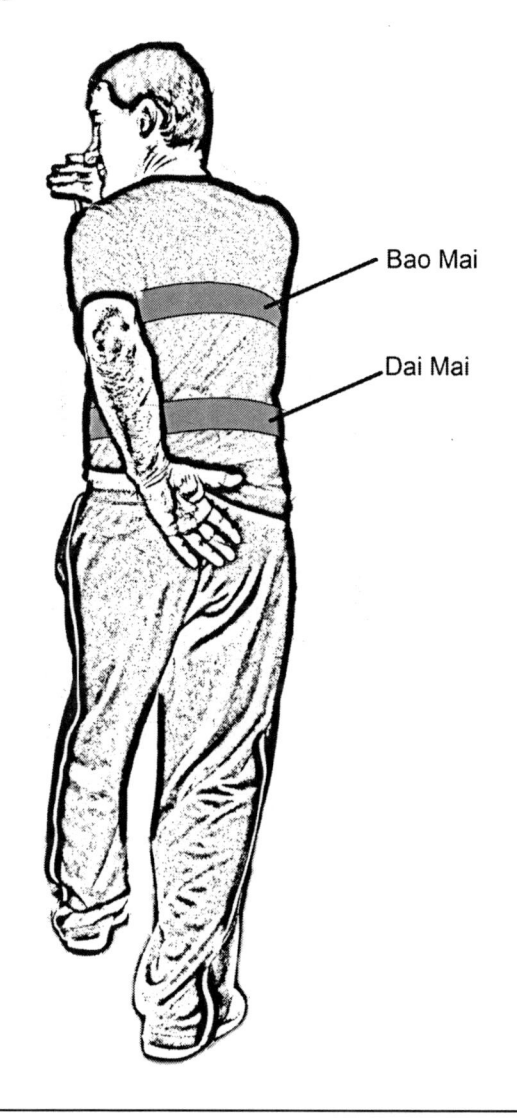

Yin Yang Fish Palm (*Yin Yang Yue Zhang*)

Opens, Stimulates & Strengthens:

- **Dai Mai (Belt Vessel)**
- **Bao Mai (Wrapper Vessel)**

Supports:

- **Lower Burner**
- **Ren Mai (Conception Vessel)**
- **Du Mai (Governing Vessel)**
- **Chong Mai (Thrusting Vessel)**

Pathways and Images

Like the Heaven Pointing Ground Drawing Palm, the Yin Yang Fish Palm creates a yin yang balance – one hand in front, one behind, one side wrapping leftward and the other wrapping rightward. The position of the arms - the inside arm which wraps behind the body and presses outward from Mingmen, and the outside arm which wraps and presses forward at about the level of the nose - effectively opens all of the acu-points that Dai Mai passes through (Mingmen (DU 4), LIV 13, GB 26, GB 27 and GB 28). The wrapping of the arms around the body also stretches and pulls Dai Mai as a whole, thereby emulating its role in wrapping around the body and the other channels.

This posture also opens the Bao Mai by the wrapping action that occurs in the chest area. Again, the arm position effectively opens and stimulates GB 22 and SP 21 and relaxes the interior and exterior aspects of the chest cavity.

Medical Qi Gong Schools teach that the Belt Channel wraps the entire body like an enveloping cocoon or a coil that spirals around the legs, torso, arms and head. The energetic hub of this vessel is at the center, where the belt channel is normally pictured.[109] The spiraling action of the body in the Yin Yang Fish Palm which comes up from the ground, passes through the torso and out into the arms is congruent with this idea that Dai Mai is a actually a series of loops that wrap the limbs and torso as imaged in the drawing below.

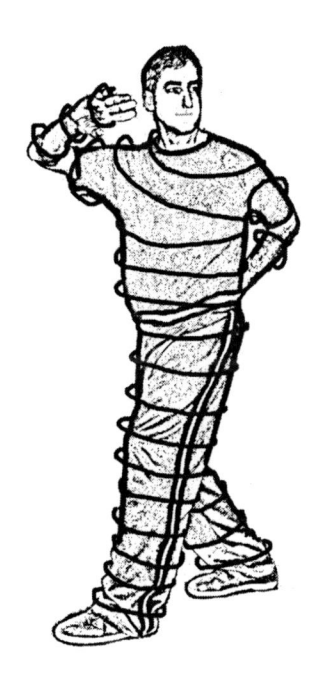

Alternative View of Dai Mai

---

[109] *Chinese Medical Qigong Therapy: A Comprehensive Clinical Text*, by Dr. Jerry Alan Johnson, PhD. D.TCM, DMQ (China). Pacific Grove, CA: The International Institute of Medical Qigong, 2000, pp.166-7.

Millstone Pushing Palm

Millstone Pushing Palm: Yin Wei & Yang Wei Mai

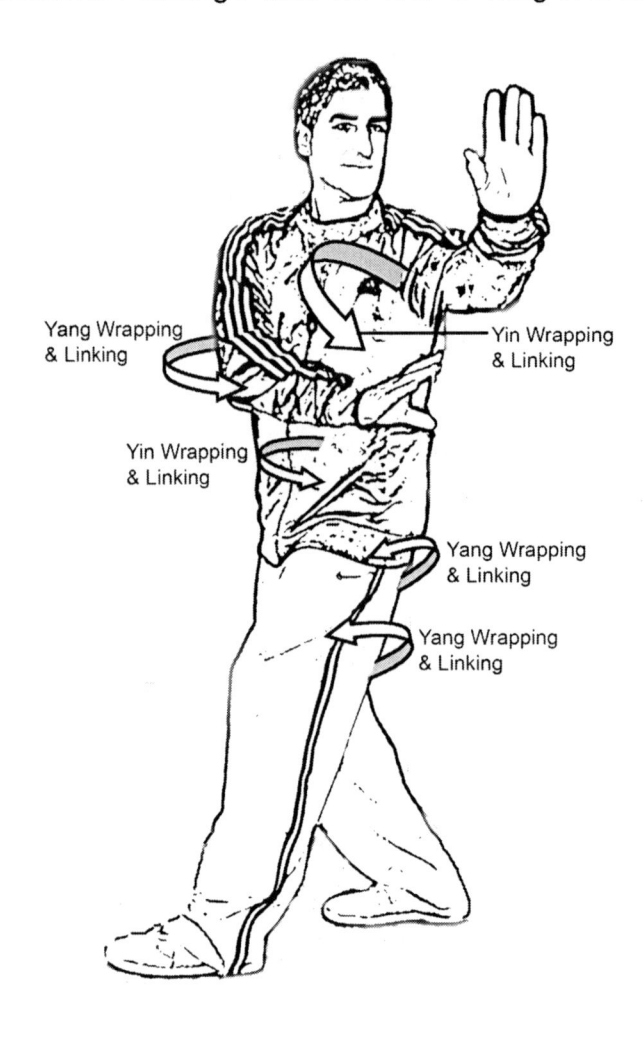

Yang Wrapping & Linking

Yin Wrapping & Linking

Yin Wrapping & Linking

Yang Wrapping & Linking

Yang Wrapping & Linking

Millstone Pushing Posture: Yang Wei Mai

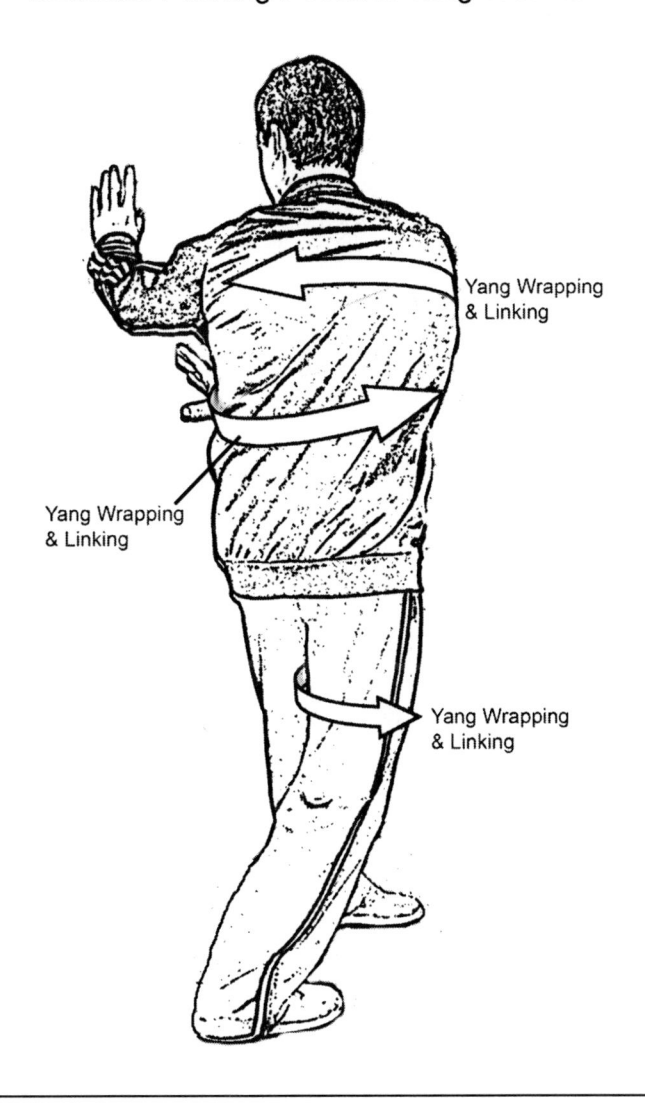

Yang Wrapping & Linking

Yang Wrapping & Linking

Yang Wrapping & Linking

Millstone Pushing Palm (*Tui Mo Zhang*)

Opens, Stimulates & Strengthens:
- **Yang Wei Mai (Yang Linking Vessel)**
- **Yin Wei Mai (Yin Linking Vessel)**

Connects Yin and Yang

Benefits and Harmonizes the Entire Body

Completes the Whole Practice

Pathways and Images

This final Ding Shi posture opens up the Wei Vessels through its folding and wrapping action. The yang surfaces of the body fold around to protect the interior yin surfaces, which in turn, gather together. This connects and harmonizes yin and yang internally and externally.

The position of the arms - wrapping inward and extending outward while the palm roots sink - engages the surplus vessels (*Yu Mai*) of the Wei Vessels and these in turn activate the master points of the Wei Vessels (P 6 and TH 5). The Millstone Pushing Palm completes the practice by connecting and linking everything that was not linked by the other postures and opening the areas of the body not opened by the other channels.

Millstone Pushing Palm: Yang Wei Mai
Alternative View

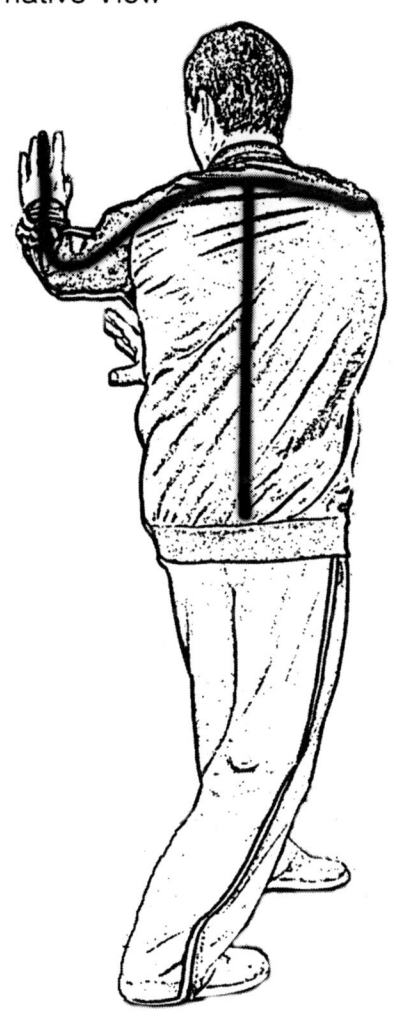

Millstone Pushing Palm
Yang Wei Mai and Yin Wei Mai: Alternative View

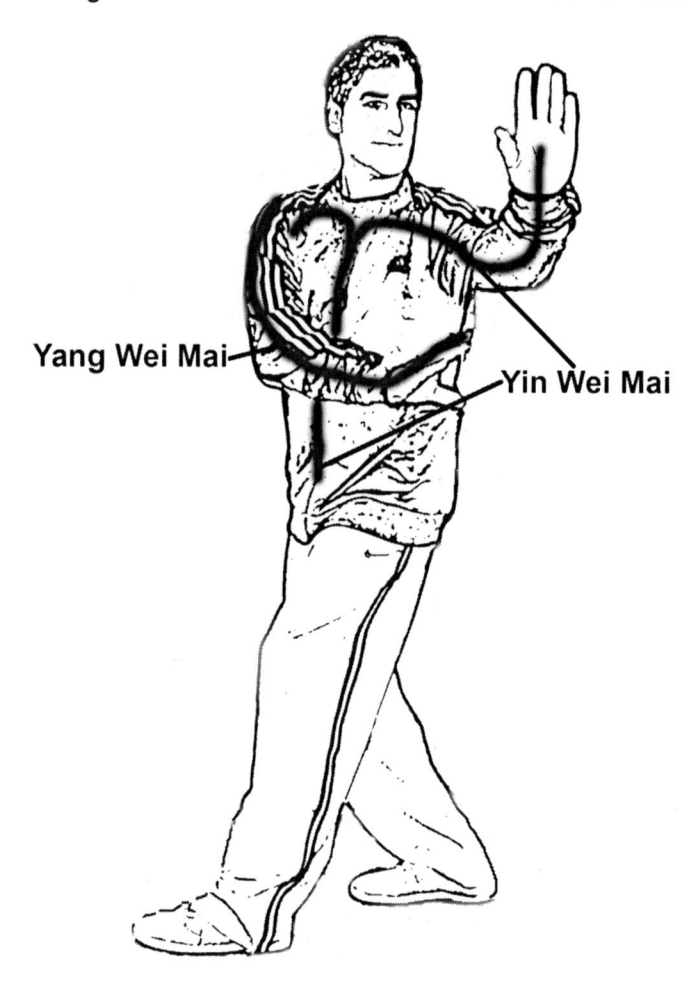

Peach Offering Palm

Peach Offering Palm: Chong Mai

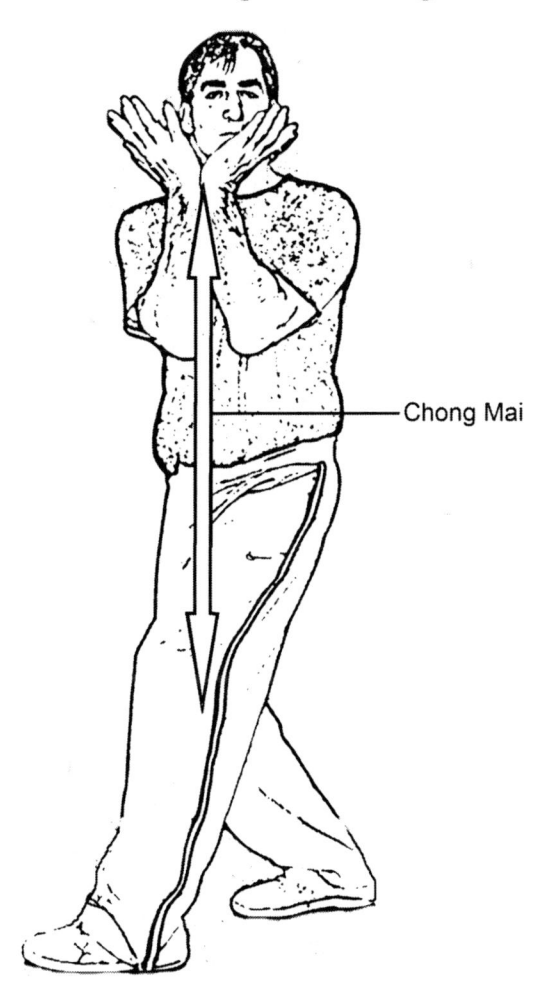

Chong Mai

Peach Offering Palm (Xian Tao Zhang)*

Stimulates Ren Mo and Du Mo
- **Expands Du Mai (yang) Outward**
- **Gathers Ren Mai (yin) Inward**

Stimulates and Opens Mingmen

Calms the Heart

Powerfully Stimulates Chong Mai
- **Connects and Inter-Transforms Kidney-Water and Heart Fire**
- **Circulates Kan-Water and Li-Fire**

Pathways and Images

    This Ding Shi posture can be used as a transitional posture in practicing Ding Shi or as a posture in its own right. The inward movement of the arms creates relative emptiness in the chest while simultaneously filling the Dantian and Mingmen. It aids in feeling the connection of the heart and kidneys, water and fire, and helps them to naturally circulate and inter-transform. The offering action of the palms helps create an upward movement along Chong Mai, while the sinking of the elbows and relaxing of the shoulders helps create a downward movement.

This palm is also called the White Ape Offers the Peach or the Double Embracing Palm. This palm is not generally part of the Ding Shi taught in Liang Zhen Pu Ba Gua and was not part of the author's discussion with Zhao Da Yuan or Li Zi Ming's notes. Therefore, the internal actions of the Peach Offering Palm as discussed here are the author's additions and viewpoints based on personal experience.

Chapter 10
Constitution and Illness: Adjusting Your Practice

Ba Gua Circle Walking Nei Gong is generally practiced as a method of strengthening the body and preventing disease. This is based on the idea that disease cannot take hold if the Jing Luo stay open and flowing. Hua Tuo, the famous Han dynasty physician expressed this as follows: *A door hinge will never become insect riddled. Rhythmic movement regulates qi, promotes digestion and blood flow and guards against disease.*[110] The practice already outlined is used by Ba Gua practitioners to prolong life, strengthen the body and prevent illness. It is also the foundation of Ba Gua Zhang the martial art. In general this is the recommended practice method as it balances and harmonizes all of the channels and collaterals. However, experienced practitioners of Ba Gua Zhang who have an understanding of Chinese medicine can alter and modify their practice in order to address imbalances and illnesses. Because this type of medical Nei Gong requires careful consideration and monitoring, **it should not be undertaken without some knowledge of Chinese medicine, especially differential diagnosis and understanding of disease etiology.** These modifications require a great deal of experience in order to be performed safely. Therefore, the concepts presented in this chapter are intended primarily to provide a complete understanding Ba Gua Circle Walking Nei Gong.

As it is impossible to cover every possible treatment, a few examples will suffice to convey the idea of how the Ba Gua Circle Walking Nei Gong can be employed to treat specific medical conditions. This discussion will be followed by a fairly complete list of signs and symptoms of channel disharmonies to help you in varying the practice of Ba Gua Circle Walking

---

[110] *Qigong Essentials of Health Promotion,* by Jiao Guorui. China Reconstructs Press, p. 11.

Nei Gong in order to address treat pathologies of the meridians. When I spoke with Zhao Da Yuan, he gave me several specific examples and told me that Li Zi Ming also gave dietary advice with each Nei Gong prescription which helped to increase the effectiveness of the Nei Gong prescription.

Sample Prescriptions

1) Tachycardia (rapid heartbeat)

Walk in the Ball Rolling Palm posture. The high hand regulates yang and the lower hand regulates yin. Focus on draining excess from the Heart and Pericardium Meridians as you walk. Let excess yang drain out of the yang palm (upper hand) and draw in yin energy with the lower hand (yin) and regulate the heartbeat. Avoid foods that activate yang like coffee, alcohol and spicy foods.

2) Bradycardia (slow heartbeat)

Walk in the Moon Holding Palm posture. Draw in yang energy through the palm centers (P 8: La Gong). Eat foods that activate the yang and tonify qi.

3) Feverish with Stiff Neck and Shoulders and No Sweating (first stage of wind-cold invasion)

Walk in the Spear Upholding Palm posture until you sweat from the upper back and chest while the lower abdomen is cool. This activates Taiyang and drives out the wind-cold which has entered the superficial layers of the body. Facilitate sweating by having rice congee with ginger and scallions. This nourishes the body and drives out cold. Do not eat rich or roasted foods.

4) Shoulder Pain

If pain is worse in the back of the shoulder, walk in the Spear Upholding Palm posture. Make sure that shoulder is relaxed. Let qi and breath move freely though the circuit of the Heart, Small Intestine, Bladder and Kidney meridians so that they are open and clear. Guide blockage and excess down from the shoulder to the feet, through the meridians.

If pain is worse in the front of the shoulder, walk in the Heaven Upholding posture in order to open and clear the Large Intestine and Stomach Meridians. Qi flows upward and outward into the hands, but also flows back inward and downward to the feet. Avoid shellfish and cold raw foods and drinks until the shoulder heals.

5) Gastric Problems, Nausea and Indigestion

Walk in the Heaven Upholding posture and relax the chest and neck so that qi can settle and naturally move downward in the Stomach Meridian. Make sure the ST 12 area is relaxed and open. Allow the organs to relax and drop downward. Eat bland, easy-to-digest food and avoid alcohol, coffee and spicy food. If the liver is involved, walk in the Moon Holding Palm and guide excess energy our through the palms while you direct the mind-intention to the area between LIV 14 and P 1 where the two Jueyin channels meet.

6) Ankle Pain and Weakness

Walk in the Heaven Pointing Ground Drawing Palm posture. Guide energy up and down the sides of the body through the two Yin Qiao Channels and the Gallbladder Meridian. Feel how the posture lifts and puts spring in the points around the ankle as energy passes from the earth upward up through the uplifted (yang) arm and pours back down to earth through the arm and hand that point downward (yin arm). If the ankle is weak and unstable, eat foods that nourish the blood and strengthen the kidneys, liver and tendons and ligaments – one classic example from Chinese dietary therapy is tendon soup.

Signs and Symptoms of Channel Disharmonies

Signs or symptoms of a channel disharmony on either the Twelve Primary Meridians and their paired Sinew Channels or on the Eight Extraordinary Channels a can generally be understood three ways:

1. The signs and symptoms stem from a blockage or disharmony in the pathway and structures that the pathway passes through.

2. The signs and symptoms stem from inappropriate functioning of the organ(s) that the pathway connects to or passes through. This relates to the Internal Branch of the pathway.

3. In the case of the Extraordinary Channels, the pathway itself has functions that can go awry.

When we consider these three possibilities it is easy to see that what appears to be an organ problem – for example frequent urination – could actually be a result of damage to a part of a meridian like the Bladder Meridian. It is also possible that ankle pain along the Bladder meridian could occur because there is an organ problem. Likewise, modifying circulation along that meridian can therefore treat either problem.

Below is a list of the signs and symptoms for the Six Axes and the Eight Extraordinary Channels. It may be helpful to review the various functions of the Zang Fu (the organs and bowels) according to Chinese medicine. This was presented earlier in Chapter Six.

Signs & Symptoms of the Six Yin-Yang Axes
Taiyang
<u>Pain and Dysfunction Along the Channel Pathway</u>

- pain at the crown
- pain at the nape

- occipital pain, stiffness
- pain at the inner canthus of the eye
- pain in scapula and back of shoulder
- inner elbow pain
- problems with the pinky
- upper back and mid-back pain and stiffness
- lower back pain and stiffness
- coccyx pain
- back of leg pain and dysfunction
- heel pain
- Achilles tendon problems
- problems with the little toe
- hemorrhoids
- clogged sinuses
- eye pain and pressure
- wind and cold causing a stiff and painful neck, nape and/or shoulders
- headache caused by wind and cold

Internal Branch Symptoms:
- diffuse abdominal pain
- urinary problems
- sinus pain and pressure in forehead area
- eye pain and pressure

Shaoyang

Pain and Dysfunction Along the Channel Pathway:
- pain in the wrist
- pain at 4th finger

- pain along outside of arm
- lateral shoulder and trapezius pain and stiffness
- sub-scapular pain
- rib sand costal pain
- side of neck tight and uncomfortable with difficulty turning the head
- temporal headache
- pain in the outer canthus of the eye
- pain in the ear
- outside of leg pain and dysfunction
- hip pain
- chronic sacro-iliac pain
- lateral ankle pain
- weak ankles
- 4th and 5th toe pain

Internal Branch Symptoms:
- stomach discomfort (gastralgia) with sour or bitter taste in mouth
- gallbladder disease: stones, cholecystitis
- bile duct problems
- fluid retention in skin and flesh
- agitation and nausea
- imbalances between the left and right sides of body

Yang Ming

Pain and Dysfunction Along the Channel Pathway:
- thumb and forefinger pain
- outside of elbow pain

- shoulder tightness, stiffness or pain
- facial pain and jaw pain
- frontal headache
- outer knee and quadriceps pain and dysfunction
- frontal ankle pain
- pain in the 2nd and 3rd toes
- sinus problems
- throat or esophagus problems
- dental problems, gums and tooth pain

Internal Branch Symptoms:
- stomach problems: reflux, indigestion, gastritis
- intestinal issues: pain, discomfort, difficult bowel movements
- pancreatic problems

Taiyin

Pain and Dysfunction Along the Channel Pathway:
- thumb pain
- wrist pain
- pain in the crease of the elbow
- shoulder pain
- medial thigh pain and weakness
- bunions
- big toe pain and stiffness

Internal Branch Symptoms:
- throat and vocal cord problems

- difficulty breathing
- bronchitis
- asthma
- frequent colds
- edema in the lower extremities
- abdominal bloating
- diarrhea
- weakness of the four limbs
- varicose veins
- chronic cough
- skin problems: eczema, psoriasis, dry skin
- respiratory problems
- menstrual and fertility problems
- lack of appetite
- reduced sense of smell and/or taste

Shaoyin

<u>Pain and Dysfunction Along the Channel Pathway</u>:
- pain in the pinky
- pain along the inside of the wrist, arm and elbow
- armpit pain and swelling
- knee pain
- tightness in the chest
- weakness of inside of lower leg
- pain and/or sensation of heat on bottom of foot

<u>Internal Branch Symptoms</u>:
- internal chill

- chilly arthritic pain
- difficulty with motivation and self-discipline
- auditory problems
- insomnia
- irregular sleep
- cold feet
- difficulty in taking a breath
- feeling frightful or fearful
- dull aching pain in low back
- achy knees
- weak low back
- decreased sex drive
- chest or heart pain

Jueyin

<u>Pain and Dysfunction Along the Channel Pathway</u>:
- painful armpit or chest
- rib and costal pain and tightness
- pain along the inside of the knee and lower leg
- groin pain
- big toe pain and dysfunction
- pain along the inside of elbow
- wrist and carpal tunnel pain
- problems with the palm of the hand
- middle finger pain and dysfunction

<u>Internal Branch Symptoms</u>:
- eye problems

- muscle spasms
- tremors
- stiff joints; muscles
- vertex headache or headache behind the eyes
- anger and quick emotional changes
- disturbances of the spirit and emotions
- palpitations; tachycardia
- chest pain; chest oppression
- high or low blood pressure
- hernia (with Taiyin)
- febrile diseases
- migraines that are worse with coffee
- diaphragmatic tightness
- menstrual pain

Signs and Symptoms of the Eight Extraordinary Channels

Du Mai

- disturbances in the yang meridians and organs
- stiff and painful neck
- low back pain on midline – can overlap with Taiyang and Yang Qiao back pain
- headache, heavy head
- vertigo
- hemorrhoids (can also be Jueyin)
- SI 3, the master point of Du Mai: used to treat, neck, shoulder and eye pain as well as acute lumbar sprain.

Ren Mai

- disturbances in the yin meridians and organs especially liver and kidney
- genital pains
- umbilical pain
- painful abdomen
- chest pain
- throat obstruction
- mouth sores
- overlaps many Chong functions
- menstruation issues
- fertility and pregnancy
- menopausal symptoms
- LU 7, the master point of Ren Mai: opens up the throat, chest and diaphragm and is used for cough and asthma.

Chong Mai

- classic Chong Mai sign: uncomfortable sensation of energy running from abdomen to chest and heart with shortness of breath
- vomiting
- heart pain, palpitations
- chest pain and tightness
- urinary and prostate problems
- sexual dysfunction
- menstrual irregularities
- infertility
- obstetric problems

- abdominal problems
- pelvic pain
- Chong Mai's role as "Sea of Blood": *When the sea of blood is in excess the person has the impression of having a large body, without any indication of disease. When it is deficient, the person has and impression of having a small body without being able to locate a disease.*[111]
- SP 4, the master point of Chong Mai: commonly used for gastric pain and vomiting, abdominal pain, pain in the spine and back pain, as well menstrual irregularity.

Dai Mai

- Classic Dai Mai Sign: feeling of being seated in cool water
- feeling of being hot above and cold below
- abdominal fullness, bloated abdomen
- weak low back
- hernias and prolapses (with Taiyin and Jueyin)
- pelvic problems
- one side of body cold or numb
- vaginal discharge
- hot or cold sensation in genitals
- urinary pain or difficulty
- GB 41, the master point of Dai Mai: sometimes used for back pain accompanied by a sense of heaviness. It is also used for pain in the lower ribs.

---

[111] *Huangdii Neijing Ling Shu: Books IV-V with commentary; Vol II.* Nguyen Van Nghi, Tran Viet Dzung, Christine Recours Nguyen. Sugar Grove, NC: Jung Tao Productions 1995 – English Edition 2006, p. 152.

Yang Wei Mai

- muscle contraction with joint stiffness
- headaches that originate at occiput on one side and go forward to same side forehead and eye[112]
- generalized aching and puffiness in lumbar area
- sacral pain that radiates to hip
- sensitivity to weather changes
- Stimulation of TH 5, the master point of Yang Wei Mai: removes obstructions in the meridians and collaterals and eliminates wind and environmental pathogens.

Yin Wei Mai

- accumulation of energy in interior of body, especially in chest and head
- thoracic pain
- abdominal pain
- cardiac pain
- diffuse headaches
- anxiety, restlessness
- palpitations
- P6, the master point of Yin Wei Mai: pacifies the stomach, calms the heart and aids circulation in the cardio-vascular system.

---

[112] *Acupuncture Energetics: A Clinical Approach for Physicians,* by Joseph M. Helms, Berkely CA: Medical Acupuncture Publishers, 1995, pp. 538-39.

Yang Qiao Mai

- one sided pain
- outer legs tight
- spasm and pain in outer leg aggravated by movement with relative flaccidity in inner leg
- can't close eyes – wide awake
- red face
- irritability
- upper back and low back pain
- shoulder pain
- BL 62, the master point of Yang Qiao Mai: can be used for problems with balance and coordination as well as sleep problems, shoulder pain and facial paralysis[113]

Yin Qiao Mai

- difficulty staying awake – can't keep eyes open
- pelvic pain
- cystitis
- irregular menses
- medial leg spasms and tightness in the inner leg with relative slackness and flaccidity in the outer leg
- Yin and Yang Qiao: difficulties with circadian rhythm and jet lag
- Kid 6, the master point of Yin Qiao Mai: can be used for a wide variety of symptoms including sore throat, insomnia, irregular menstruation and urinary problems.

---

[113] *Applied Channel Theory in Chinese Medicine: Wang Ju-Yi's Lectures on Channel Therapeutics* by Wang Ju-Yi and Jason Robertson Seattle: Eastland Press, 2008, p. 303.

Chapter 11
Advanced Walking Patterns

Once you are proficient in the basic Ba Gua Circle Walking Nei Gong, you can move on to more advanced methods of stepping. Three of these methods are outlined below. All three stepping methods can be performed with any of the nine postures previously discussed. Once one is proficient with the stepping and postures, they may be freely interchanged.

Figure Eight Pattern

This is essentially two connected circles. In the picture below the figure on the right is walking clockwise in the right Millstone Pushing Palm posture. When he reaches the intersection of the two circles, he "changes" by taking a left swing step (bai bu) onto the left hand circle. Simultaneously, the body swings to the left so that he is now walking counter-clockwise in the left Millstone Pushing Palm posture. He then continues clockwise until he reaches the intersection of the two circles and uses a right bai bu step to walk clockwise again on the original circle.

Figure 8 Walking Pattern

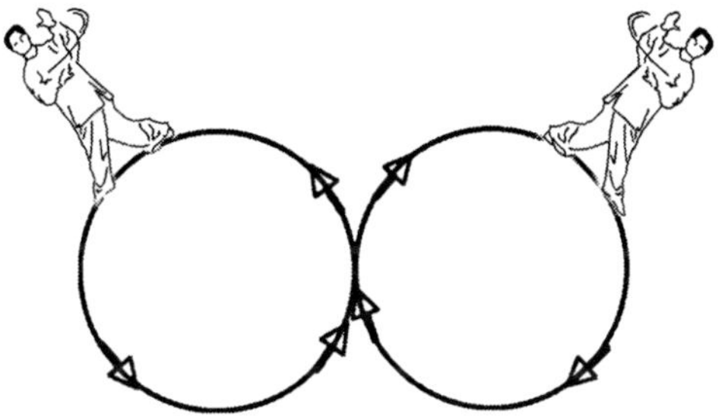

This method of walking can be used for any and all of the eight Ding Shi Palms. One can walk around one circle several times or for several minutes before switching to the other circle, or you can change each time you come to where the two circles intersect. You can also try walking on different size circles - for example a circle that takes 6 or 8 steps to complete or a larger circle that takes 12 or 16 steps to complete. This practice method adds the element of smoothly changing directions by moving onto a different circle. It makes you focus on the palms and the steps in a different way. The figure eight walking method can then be extrapolated to the nine palace walking method which uses nine circles. Traditionally, practitioners used two posts or two trees to fix the points at the centers of the circles.

The Yin Yang Winding Step: Method #1

This stepping pattern employs the image of the yin-yang diagram, sometimes known as the yin-yang fish. In this method you walk through the center of the circle following the curving line that separates the two fish that make up the yin yang diagram. When walking counterclockwise the center line is traversed as follows:

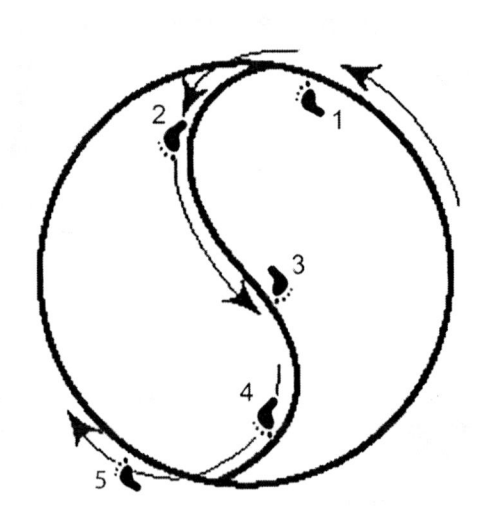

Steps 1 and 2

As you approach the head of the fish on the right, the right foot hooks (kou bu) in order to step onto the center line.

Step 3

Then the left performs a swing step (bai bu) along the center line. The body holds the same posture and winds to the left.

Step 4

This is followed by a right bai bu, along the center line as the body and the hands swing toward the right.

Step 5

A final kou bu with the left brings you back onto the perimeter of the circle, this time walking clockwise. The body continues to turn rightward as you walk the circle.

To Reverse Direction:

Perform the four-step turn (Chapter Five) on the periphery of the circle and walk counterclockwise again. One can walk one or more circles before executing the direction changes.

The Yin Yang Winding Step: Method #2

Another method of performing the Yin Yang Winding Step is to change direction by making a very tight Kou Bu (hook step) into the tail of the fish. Start by walking counterclockwise.

1. Change direction as you approach the tail of the black fish using a tight right hook step (Kou Bu). The body turns leftward.
2. The left foot swings (Bai Bu) to walk along the center line separating the two fish, but as it settles into the floor, it hooks (Kou) slightly, and the body turns all the way left.

3. The right foot hooks (Kou Bu) to walk along the head of the black fish as the body turns to the right and the hands swing rightward).
4. The left foot swings (Bai Bu) as you approach the tip of tail of the white fish and the body and hands begin to swing back leftward.
5. The body continues to turn leftward as the right foot hooks, to bring you back on to the circle so that you are again walking counterclockwise.

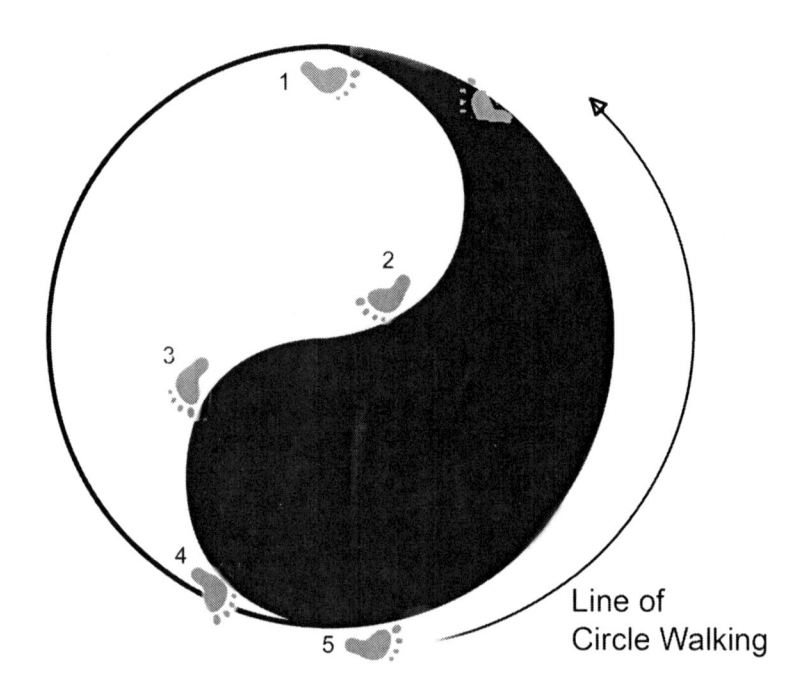

Counterclockwise Yin-Yang Winding Step

Line of Circle Walking

When holding the last five Ding Shi postures - Ball Holding Palm, Spear Holding Palm, Heaven Pointing and Ground Drawing Palm, Yin Yang Fish Palm and the Millstone Pushing Palm - you will need to swing the arms to change to the other side as you move into the step 3, and then change again as you move through steps 4 and 5.

6. **Now Reverse Direction** using the four-step turn (Chapter Five) on the periphery of the circle in order to walk clockwise. Walk clockwise for several circles.
7. Then mentally flip the diagram horizontally as shown below. This will allow you to execute the same winding step, entering the middle line from a clockwise direction.

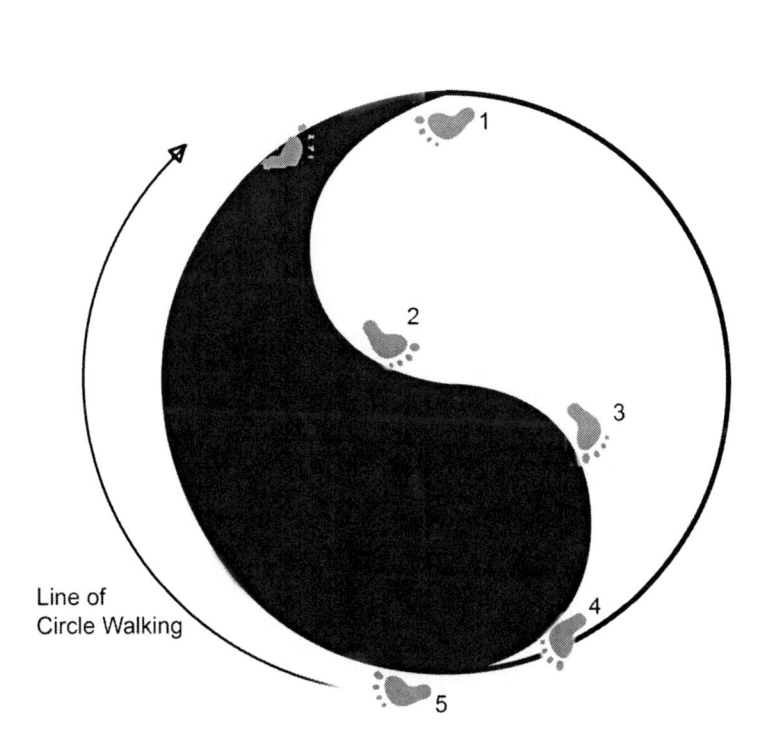

Clockwise Yin-Yang Winding Step

Once again you will exit onto the periphery of the circle, still walking clockwise. **Reverse Direction** using the four step turn Chapter Five) on the periphery of the circle in order to again walk counterclockwise.

Although these changes can be made freely, one balanced practice method using Yin Yang Winding Step Method #2 is as follows:

1. walk a full circle counterclockwise.

2. walk the yin yang winding line through the center of the circle starting at the tail of the black fish.
3. walk a half-circle counterclockwise and change direction using the four-step turn (Chapter Five) or the alternative turning method (Chapter 6).
4. walk a full circle clockwise.
5. walk the yin yang winding line through the center of the circle starting at the tail of the white fish.
6. walk a half-circle clockwise and change direction to walk counterclockwise again.

This pattern can be repeated indefinitely and with all the Ding Shi postures.

Nine Palace Circle Walking Pattern

This walking method is based on a the arrangement of the Post-Heaven arrangement of the *Yi Jing* trigrams. Daoist shamanic priests traditionally walked this pattern relating to the dipper constellation in order to ritually harmonize with the heavens. This pattern also creates a "magic square," in which the three numbers add up to 15 in any direction.

4	9	2
3	5	7
8	1	6

The nine-palace pattern is depicted below. In the practice of Ba Gua Circle Walking Nei Gong, one walks around nine posts in the ground so that one is moving through a series of nine interconnected circles. Many of us who live in apartments do not have a yard in which we can sink nine posts, so you can put nine paper cups on the floor with numbers written on them to better help you visualize the pattern. Later you can simply imagine the nine posts or nine circles.

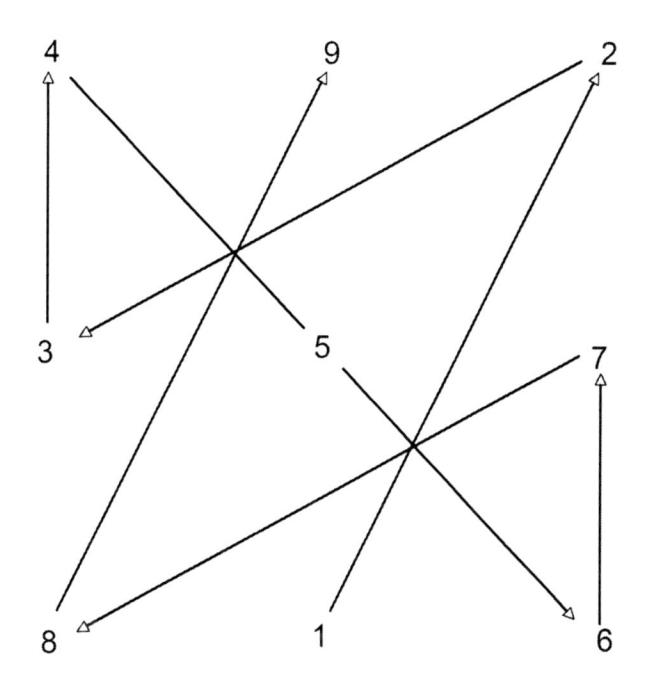

Sequence of the Nine Palaces According to the Numbers of the Magic Square

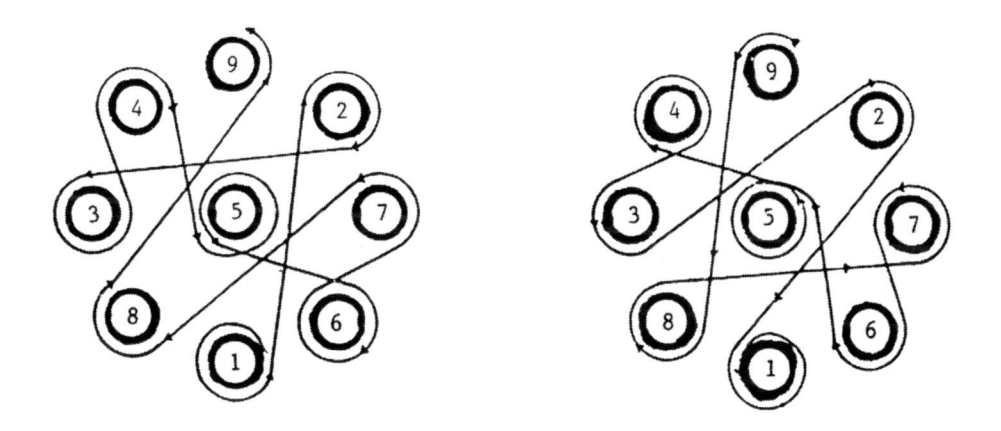

There are many ways to walk the nine palaces. The basic method is to follow the pattern shown in the diagrams above. The simplest and most effective way to do this is to walk a complete circle around one post. Then walk a circle around the central post (#5) before moving on to the next post.

1. Start by walking counterclockwise around post #1.
2. When you intersect its connecting point with post #5 step onto that circle, now walking clockwise.
3. After circling post # 5, change to walk counterclockwise around post #2.

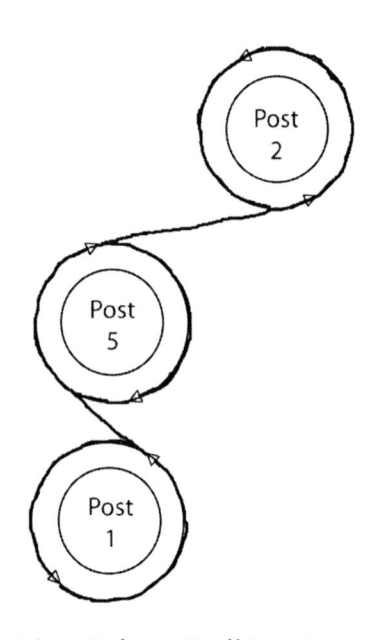

Nine Palace Walking 1

4. After walking around counterclockwise around post #2, return to post #5, circling clockwise.
5. From post #5, change to walk counterclockwise around post #3.

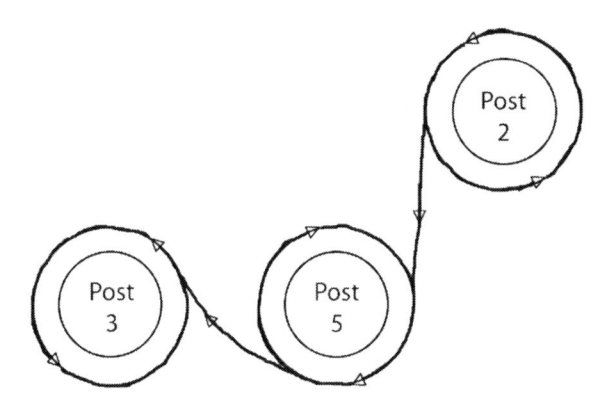

Nine Palace Walking 2

6. After circling post #3, return to walk clockwise around post #5.
7. From post #5 change to walk counterclockwise around post #4.

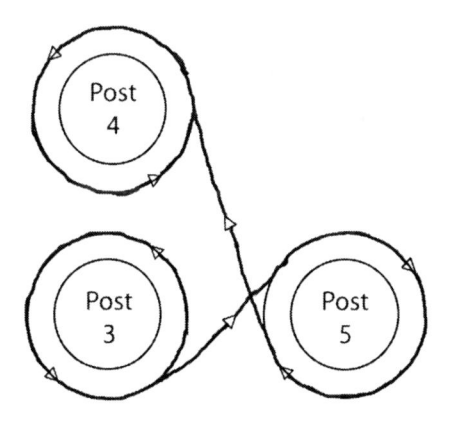

Nine Palace Walking 3

8. Continue to walk this way until you reach post #9 and then you can reverse the direction going from post #9 sequentially back to post #1.

Essentially this is just a fancy version of the figure-eight stepping pattern, but it emphasizes the eight directions and varies the changes so the mind has to stay alert to make the steps. There is no rule about how many times you circle a single post, how you change the palms or when to change them. However, an interesting and challenging practice method is to walk sequentially from post #1 to post #9 and back to post #1 again using the Downward Sinking Palm. Make at least one circle around each post. Then do the same with each of the other 7 palms.

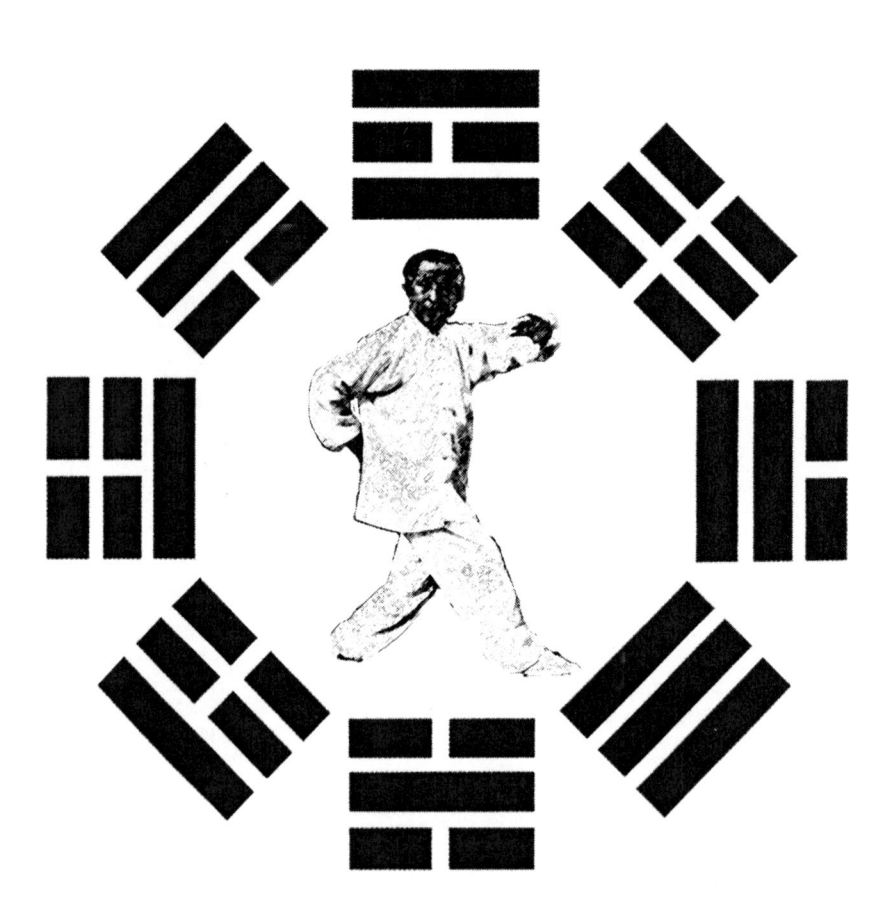

Chapter 12
The Ba Gua Zhang Energy Accepting Palm

The Healing Power of Trees and Plants

The healing power of trees and plants is indisputable. In China there is a saying: "whoever loves flowers lives long."[114] Living among trees and plants calms and relaxes the body. Even just taking a walk in the woods can make us feel better. In city environments, trees and plants help to reduce pollutants in the air that can trigger respiratory allergies such as asthma. In a recent study, abdominal surgery patients staying in rooms with plants had a faster recovery, lower anxiety levels and took less medication that those that had no plants in their rooms.[115] Laboratory and clinical investigations have found that viewing natural settings can create significant positive changes in blood pressure, heart activity, muscle tension and brain electrical activity.[116] Proximity to nature also effectively lowered activity in the sympathetic nervous system and produced substantial recuperation in the psychological component of stress. People exposed to natural settings with plants and trees, as opposed to built-up environments, had lower levels of fear and anger, and also reported much higher levels of positive feelings.[117] In a another study, subjects were exposed to stress by either driving through urban traffic or taking a series of difficult tests. Recovery from stress, measured through both blood pressure data and emotional self-reports, indicated that *recovery was appreciably greater if persons looked at a nature*

---

[114] *The Mystery of Longevity,* By Liu Zhengcai. Beijing: Foreign Language Press 1990 and 1996, p. 70.
[115] http://www.types-of-flowers.org/blog/flowers-have-healing-benefits/
[116] *Health Benefits of Gardens in Hospitals,* by Roger S. Ulrich, Ph.D. Paper for conference: *Plants for People,* International Exhibition Floriade 2002
Center for Health Systems and Design -Colleges of Architecture and Medicine
Texas A & M University, p. 3.
[117] Ibid, p. 4.

setting dominated by vegetation rather than a built environment without nature.[118]

In China, proximity to different trees, plants and flowers has long been known to produce specific therapeutic effects. For example, geraniums calm the body, dissipate fatigue and induce sleep. Having two pots of geraniums in the bedroom can help you to fall asleep quickly.[119] Trees help the body replenish qi, remove stagnation from the meridians and calm the spirit. Bushes are similar, but are not as powerful in this regard as trees. Flowers affect the spirit, emotions and nervous system. The various colors and scents of flowers also play a role in their effects on the qi.

Ba Gua practitioners often practice the Circle Walking Nei Gong around a tree. There are several reasons for this. The tree can serve as the center of the circle and a focal point for the gaze and intention. The tree can also be used to replenish the qi, strengthen the body and the organs and dispel pathogenic qi. The tree most commonly combined with Neigong and meditative practices is the pine. Pine trees are considered to be yang and to promote longevity. They replenish and activate the qi. Pine trees home to the liver, can disperse blockages in the meridians and help the tendons to feel comfortable and relaxed. While trees in general tend to home to the spleen and stomach because they are literally rooted in the earth, and to the liver because they are emblematic of liver-wood energy, some distinctions can be made. The list below is by no means exhaustive.

Properties of Trees:

- Pine trees home to the Liver
- Apple trees home to the Heart

---

[118] Ibid.
[119] *The Mystery of Longevity,* By Liu Zhengcai, p. 69.

- Willow trees home to the Spleen
- Poplar trees home to the Lung
- Cypress trees home to the Kidney
- Locust trees clear internal heat and balance the Heart
- Birch trees home to the Spleen, Stomach and Intestines – they help clear dampness
- Ginkgo trees home to the Lung and help with skin problems
- Plum trees home to the Spleen and Stomach
- Hawthorn trees aid digestion and blood pressure
- Elm trees calm the mind and strengthen the stomach
- Bamboo homes to the Liver, Gallbladder and Heart

Properties of Flowers:
- Lotus Flowers: beneficial for the Heart
- Rugosa Rose: beneficial for the Heart
- Jasmine: regulates circulation of qi; relaxes and calms spirit
- Lilac: purifies the air and kills bacteria
- Cape Jasmine: helps Liver and Gallbladder; hepatitis; cholecystitis
- Geranium: calming; dissipates fatigue and induces sleep.

The Ba Gua Energy Accepting Palm

This is a method of practicing Ba Gua Circle Walking Nei Gong in which you absorb the energy of a tree through your palms as you walk around it. Potted plants or flowers can also be used for this purpose, particularly in city environments where circle walking around a tree might not be practical. To understand this practice, it is important to know that in Chinese medical theory, there are considered to be three levels in nature and in the body that connect to three important acupuncture points. These points are also sometimes referred to as "Dantian", in the sense that Dantian is not only the area below the navel, but more generally can refer to a place where qi gathers.

The Three Levels (Three Dan Tian)

1. Heaven   DU 20   Bai Hui ("Hundred Meetings")
2. Humans   REN 17   Dan Zhong ("Chest Center")
3. Earth   KID 1   Yong Quan ("Bubbling Well")

The yang energy of heaven passes into the body at the vertex (DU 20), and moves downward to connect with KID 1 (at the sole of the foot) and earth. The yin energy of earth enters at KID 1 and moves upward to connect with DU 20 and heaven. These energies connect at both Dantian (below the navel), the "Lower Sea of Qi" and REN 17, the chest center, also called the "Upper Sea of Qi." REN 17 in turn connects with the Pericardium Meridian and Lao Gong (P 8 – "Palace of Labor"). Lao Gong lies in the center of the palm. From Lao Gong we can take in, or accept energy from living things.

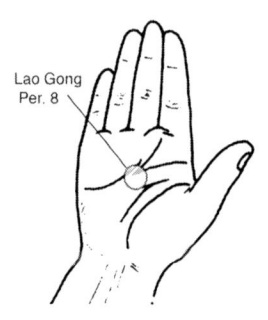

In Ba Gua, the Energy Accepting Palm is based on the Eight Ding Shi postures and their ability to open and balance the Jing Luo. This is combined with an understanding of the healing properties of plants, trees, and flowers. For example, while walking around a pine tree in the Moon Holding Palm, which opens Jueyin and Taiyin, you can draw in the qi from the pine through your palms in order help calm the heart and pericardium, open the meridians, nourish the liver and relax the tendons. Some postures can be slightly modified to face the Lao Gong acu-point toward the tree. With the Heaven Upholding Palm, qi can be drawn in from the hanging branches of the tree. This might be helpful for dispelling dampness and strengthening the spleen, stomach and intestines. With the Downward Sinking Palm, qi can be drawn in from the roots in the ground around the tree. Walking around a pine tree in the Downward Sinking Palm posture and drawing energy up from the roots can help to stimulate circulation in Ren Mai and Du Mai.

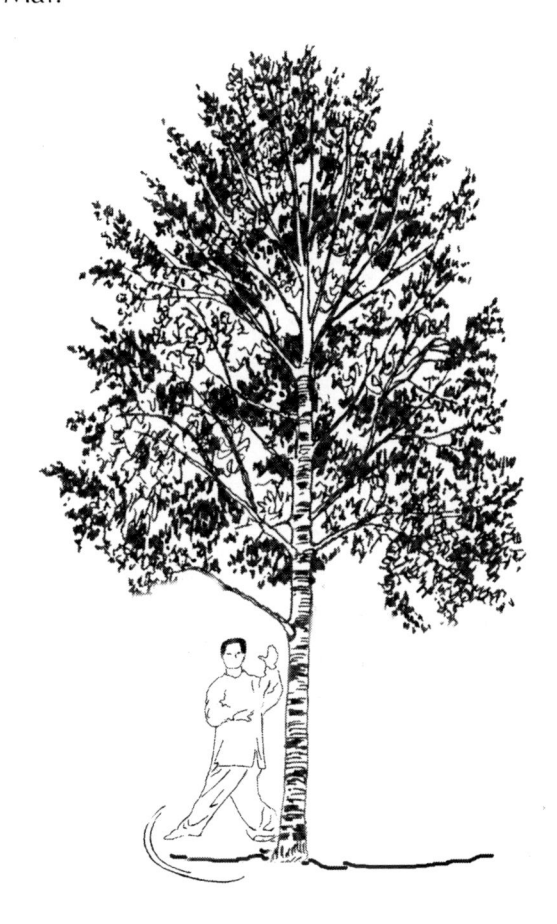

In the Heaven Pointing Ground Drawing Palm, the palm of the upper hand is turned to face forward, so that it can better accept energy form the tree or plant. This is a variation of the Heaven Pointing Ground Drawing Palm practiced by many of Li Zi Ming's Students. This variation is pictured below.

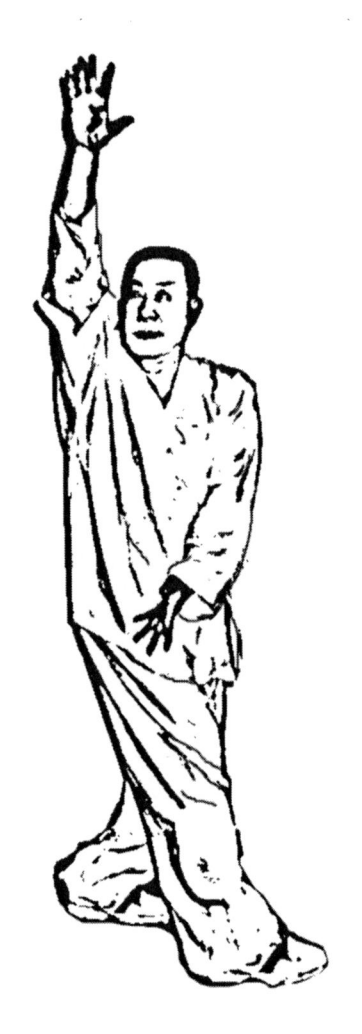

Drawing from an author photo of Zhang Hua Sen

Even though we are focusing on qi being accepted and absorbed by our palms, qi is simultaneously being absorbed through our crown (DU 20) and the soles of our feet (KID 1). Once you are accustomed to accepting the qi of the tree through your palms you can also feel it coming up from the ground through the soles and through the body to the vertex. From DU 20, qi then moves up into the branches of the tree, flows down the trunk and into the roots to come up again through your feet. You become part of the circuit of energy which flows through the tree and now through you. This circulation of qi can also be reversed – the qi pouring from the branches of the tree into the crown of your head and down the body into the feet and then into the ground, into the roots of the tree, and up the trunk again to the branches.

End this kind of practice by standing still with the eyes half closed. Feel your connection with the tree, the earth and the heavens for a minute or two in order to complete your practice.

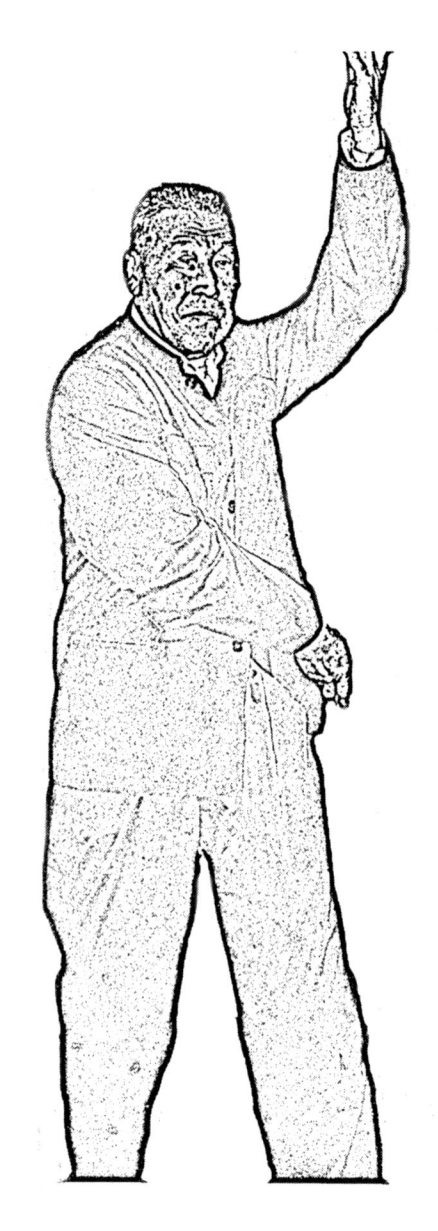

Heaven Pointing Ground Drawing Palm
Drawing from an author photo of Wang Shi Tong

Bibliography

A Brief Introduction to the Body Strengthening Function of the Eight Diagram Palm Qi Gong by Li Zi Ming, Translated by Huang Guo Qi, Pa Kua Chang Journal Vol. 5 No. 1 Nov./Dec. 1994, Pacific Grove CA: High View Publications pp. 17-19.

Acupuncture Energetics: A Clinical Approach for Physicians, by Joseph M. Helms, Berkely CA: Medical Acupuncture Publishers, 1995.

Additional Comments to Passage 3:3 in the Zhuangzi, by Brook Ziporyn http://hackettpublishing.com/zhuangzi3.3

Anatomical Roots of Chinese Medicine and Acupuncture by Claus C. Schnorrenberger (After a lecture presented to the British Medical Acupuncture Society, University of Warwick, England, BMAS Spring Meeting 2006.

An Exposition of the Extraordinary Vessels: Acupuncture, alchemy & Internal Medicine by Charles Chace and Miki Shima. Seattle: Eastland Press, 2010.

Anti-Aging Benefits of Qigong, by Kenneth Sancier PhD., http://www.qigonginstitute.org/html/papers/Anti-Aging_Benefits_of_Qigong.html

Applied Channel Theory in Chinese Medicine: Wang Ju-Yi's Lectures on Channel Therapeutics by Wang Ju-Yi and Jason Robertson Seattle: Eastland Press, 2008.

Atlas of Acupuncture by Claudia Focks. Churchill Livingstone (Elsevier Limited), 2008.

Ba Gua Zhang, by Jiang Rong-Qiao, translated by Huang Guo Qi and Tom Bisio.

Celestial Lancets: A History and Rationale of Acupuncture and Moxa, by Lu Gwei-Djen and Joseph Needham. First published by Cambridge University Press in 1980. Routledge Curzon reprint in 2002.

Channel Systems of Chinese Medicine: the Eight Extraordinary Vessels Lecture by Jeffery C. Yuen April 12 -13 2003. Copyright New England School of Acupuncture & Jeffrey C. Yuen. 2005.

Chinese Medical Qigong Therapy: A Comprehensive Clinical Text, by Dr. Jerry Alan Johnson PhD. D.TCM, DMQ (China). Pacific Grove, CA: The International Institute of Medical Qigong, 2000.

Chuang Tzu: Basic Writings, translated by Burton Watson New York: Columbia University Press, 1964.

Chinese Acupuncture and Moxibustion (Revised Edition) Chief Editor Cheng Xinnong, Beijing: Foreign Language Press, 1999.

Chinese Healing Exercises by Livia Kohn, Honolulu: University of Hawai'i Press, 2008.

Chuang Tzu: The Inner Chapters, translated by A.C. Graham. Indianapolis, Indiana: Hackett Publishing Co. Inc., 1981, 2002.

Classical Baguazhang volume XIII: Sun Style Baguazhang (Ba Gua Quan Xie and Bagua Jian Xue) by Sun Lutang. Translated by Joseph Crandall Smiling Tiger Martial Arts: Pinole CA. 2002.

Core Patterns of The Shang Han Lung: Part I. Lecture by Arnaud Versluys. Pacific College of Oriental Medicine in NYC, 2009.

Early Chinese Medical Literature: The Mawangdui Manuscripts, Translation and Study by Donald Harper. London and New York: Kegan Paul International, 1998.

Effects of Qigong Therapy on Arthritis: A Review and Report of a Pilot Trial by Kevin W Chen and Tianjun Liu. Medical Paradigm: June 2004 - Volume 1, Number 1.; www.wishus.org/researchpapers/Arthritis.pdf

Grasping the Wind: An Exploration into the Meaning of Chinese Acupuncture Point Names. Andrew Ellis, Nigel Wiseman, Ken Boss. Brookline, MA: Paradigm Press, 1989.

Health Benefits of Gardens in Hospitals, by Roger S. Ulrich, Ph.D. Paper for conference: *Plants for People,* International Exhibition Floriade 2002

Center for Health Systems and Design -Colleges of Architecture and Medicine,Texas A & M University.

How Meditation May Change the Brain, by Sindya N. Bhanoo January 28, 2011, New York Times http://well.blogs.nytimes.com/2011/01/28/how-meditation-may-change-the-brain/

Huangdii Neijing Ling Shu: Books IV-V with commentary; Vol II. Nguyen Van Nghi, Tran Viet Dzung, Christine Recours Nguyen. Sugar Grove, NC: Jung Tao Productions 1995 – English Edition 2006.

Liang Chen-P'u's "Old Eight Palms" Pa Kua Chang Journal Vol.3, No. 3 March/April 1993. Pacific Grove, CA: High View Publications.

Liang Zhen Pu Eight Diagram Palm by Li Zi Ming; translated by Huang Guo Qi and compiled and edited by Vince Black. Pacific Grove, CA: High View Publications, 1993, p. 21.

*Ligamentous Articular Strain: Osteopathic Manipulative Techniques for the Body,*by Conrad A. Speece, D.O. and William Thomas Crow, D.O., Seattle: Eastland Press, 2001.

Ling Shu or The Spiritual Pivot, Translated by Wu Jing-Nuan. The Taoist Center, Washington DC, 1993, 2002, 2004, Distributed by University of Hawai'I Press.

Multifaceted Health Benefits of Medical Qigong, by Kenneth M. Sancier, Ph.D. and Devatara Holman MS, MA, Lac J. Alt Compl Med. 2004; 10(1):163-166.

Nan Ching: the Classic of Difficulties, translated and annotated by Paul U. Unschuld. Berkely: University of California Press, 1986.

Nei Gong: The Authentic Classic – A Translation of the Nei Gong Zhen Chuan, translated by Tom Bisio, Huang Guo-Qi and Joshua Paynter. Outskirts Press Inc, 2011.

Neuroanatomic Basis of Acupuncture Points, by Ying Xia, Fei Zhou, Dengkai Huang (2010 from *Acupuncture Therapy for Neurological Diseases.* Springer p.53 ISBN 9783642108556,
http://en.wikipedia.org/wiki/Acupuncture_point

Ba Gua Chang Journal Vol.6, No. 1 Nov/Dec 1995. Pacific Grove, CA: High View Publications.

Qigong Essentials of Health Promotion, by Jiao Guorui. China Reconstructs Press.

Qigong Reduced Blood Pressure and Catecholamine Levels of Patients with Essential Hypertension, by Myung-Suk Lee, Myeong Soo Lee et als 2003, Vol. 113, No. 12, Pages 1691-1701.
http://informahealthcare.com/doi/abs/10.1080/00207450390245306

Relationship of Acupuncture Points and Meridians to Connective Tissue Planes, by Helene M. Langevin and Jason A. Yandow. The Anatomical Record (New Aant.) 269:257–265, 2002.

Science of Internal Strength Boxing, by Zhang Nai Qi (1933). Translated by Marcus Brinkman Taipei, Taiwan, 2005.

Tai Chi Reported to Ease Fibromyalgia, by Pam Belluck. The New York Times, August 18, 2010.
http://www.nytimes.com/2010/08/19/health/19taichi.html

Taoist Yoga: Alchemy & Immortality by Lu K'uan Yu (Charles Luk). Maine: Samuel Weiser, Inc. 1973.

The Acupuncturist's Clinical Handbook, by Jeffrey H. Jacob, D.O.M., L.Ac New York: Integrative Wellness Inc. 2003; Sante Fe: Aesclipius Press 1996.

The *Amazing Fascial Web, Part I,* By Leon Chaitow, ND, DO. *Massage Today* May, 2005, Vol. 05, Issue 05.

The Attacking Hands of Ba Gua Zhang, by Gao Ji Wu with Tom Bisio, photos by Valerie Ghent. New York: Trip Tych enterprises LLC, 2010.

The Eight Extraordinary Meridians, by Claude Larre and Eisabeth Rochat de la Vallee. Monkey Press 1997.

The Essentials of Ba Gua Zhang, by Gao Ji-Wu and Tom Bisio, Photographs by Valerie Ghent. New York: Trip Tych Enterprises LLC, 2007.

The Extraordinary Acupuncture Meridians: Homeostatic Vessels By Leon I. Hammer, MD. First published in the American Journal of Acupuncture, Vol. 8, No. 2, June 1980.

The Mystery of Longevity, By Liu Zhengcai. Beijing: Foreign Language Press1990 and 1996.

The Origins of Pa Kua Chang - Part 3, by Dan Miller. Pa Kua Chang Journal Vol. 3, No. 4 May/June 1993. Pacific Grove, CA: High View Publications, p. 27.

The Penetrating Vessel by Giovanni Maciocia, First published in NZRA Journal of TCM, Winter 2006.

The Relaxation Response, By Herbert Benson MD, New York: HarperCollins, 2000. First Published in 1975 by William Morrow and Co. Inc.

The Science of Internal Strength Training by Zhang Nai Qi (1933). Translated by Marcus Brinkman. Insiderasia.com, 2005.

The Secondary Vessels of Acupuncture: A Detailed Account of their Energies, Meridians and Control Points by Royston Low. New York: Thorsons Publishers Inc. 1983.

The Taoist Body by Kristofer Schipper - Berkely, Los Angeles: University of California Press 1993.

Visceral Manipulation by John Pierre Barral and Philip Mercier. Seattle: Eastland Press: 1988.

Vital Nourishment: Departing From Happiness by Francois Jullien, translated by Arthur Goldhammer. New York: Zone Books, 2007.

Walking Compared With Vigorous Exercise for the Prevention of Cardiovascular Events in Women by Joanne Manson, M.dD, Dr P.H., Philip Greenland, M.D., et als New England Journal of Medicine 2002 Vol. 347, No. 10 · September 5, 2002 · www.nejm.org

Wei Tuo Qi Gong – Climbing the Mountain: The Essence of Qi Gong and Martial Arts, by Jonathan Snowiss. Xlibris, 2010.

What's the Single Best Exercise? by Gretchen Reynolds Published: April 15, 2011 New York Times Magazine
ttp://www.nytimes.com/2011/04/17/magazine/mag-17exercise-t.html

Yellow Emperor's Canon of Internal Medicine, Bing Wang, translated by Nelson Liansheng Wu and Andrew Qi Wu. China Science and Technology Press.

Zang Fu: The Organ Systems of Traditional Chinese Medicine 2nd Edition by Jeremy Ross London: Churchill Livingstone, 1985 pp. 9-10.

Zhuangzi: The Essential Writings with Selections from Traditional Commentaries, translated by Brook Ziporyn. Indianapolis IN: Hackett Publishing Co., 2009.

Other Books by Outskirts Press

Available from Outskirts Press:
http://outskirtspress.com/bookstore/

Nei Gong: The Authentic Classic
A Translation of the Nei Gong Zhen Chuan

translated by Tom Bisio, Huang Guo-Qi and Joshua Paynter

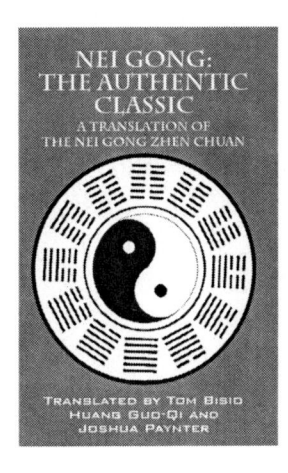

Mr. Bisio has crafted something which sits at the intersection of the scholarly and the practical: it will certainly aid martial/internal artists with alignments and combat strategy, while readers interested in the esoteric side of the internal arts will gain access into the alchemy that is present in these practices and Yi Jing scholars may find a very useful and different take on interpretation of the trigrams.

-amazon.com Review

The book is an invaluable supplement to training with a teacher and may bridge many gaps and questions marks for students in regard to structure, shen fa, fa jing/fa li and issuing, intent, san ti shi and many other difficult to grasp concepts in the art, strategy and medicinal attributes and applications of nei gong, in particular for students of Xing yi, yet valuable to an open minded student of any internal art. This classic can also serve as indispensable tool to teachers in order to help articulate difficult ideas in a new light, or as a companion guide and as part of an essential reading list and resource to students outside of actual practice. As one's knowledge of the art expands, the value of this text/translation will increase over the years.

-amazon.com Review

Strategy and Change: An Examination of Military Strategy, the I-Ching and Ba Gua Zhang by Tom Bisio

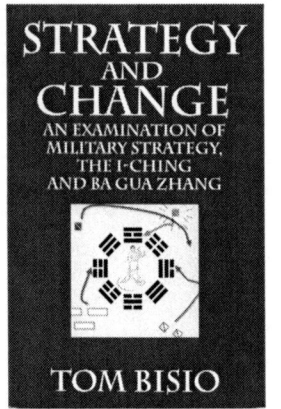

What is remarkable about Tom Bisio's approach to Ba Gua Zhang, as exemplified in Strategy and Change, is his lucid and pragmatic explication of the relationship of internal energy and body states to external situations of crisis. His approach is holistic, not linear, so one can enter this book at any point and find insight. By relating internal flow of energy to external battle plans from military thinkers as diverse as Sun Tzu to Mao Ze Dong and Belisarius to Clausewitz, Strategy and Change offers numerous examples of how spontaneously deploying internalized strategies consistently overcomes traditional martial maneuvers. For me, the real benefit of this book is its application to the strategic moments we all face daily, of holding and releasing power in the body with mindfulness, whether negotiating in business, competing in sports, disciplining one's self (or one's kids!), or any circumstance where one's self goes out into the world with intent, not necessarily to conquer but to persuade and prevail without resentment or backlash. I highly recommend this book of strategy, which so compellingly demonstrates the Daoist principles of transforming conflict into creative tension and the emotional resolution and satisfaction of achieving victories that free us to move forward by leaving behind only the soft echo of self.

-amazon.com Review

This is an in-depth contemplation on the meaning of strategy with a wealth of examples from both Western and Eastern Military history. Using such sources as Sun Zi, Liddel, Francoise Jullien, and our own Kang Ge Wu, the author shows many correlates between martial arts and the wide ranging application of strategy in both war and daily life. We share many of Mr. Bisio's views and have also had Bagua instructors who see little correlation between the I Ching, for example, and the concepts of Bagua in actual practice. However, we feel there is a wider activity here than one may first suspect. Asians, long familiar with these sources, already think along these strategic avenues. But as Kung Fu becomes a shared art in the world, the original source materials bear investigation. It's not a matter so much of keeping alive the thoughts of previous generations as examining the underpinnings of the most basic ideas. Tom Bisio supplies many examples from famous military histories: Hannibal to Cao Cao, then correlates them to martial arts examples which add life and immediacy to the concepts. Like

Musashi, we can see the connection between beating one man and employing ten thousand troops. He takes these examples and correlates them to that mysterious and perennial source of wisdom, the I-Ching. Should start some people thinking and the stories, mostly unknown to non-Asians, are the very stuff of the martial inheritance.
    -Ted Mancuso Plum Publications (plumpub.com)